I dedicate this book to every first-time flyer who trusted
a stranger by saying "Yes!" to the seemingly strange
question, "Wanna fly?"

MOVE, CONNECT, PLAY

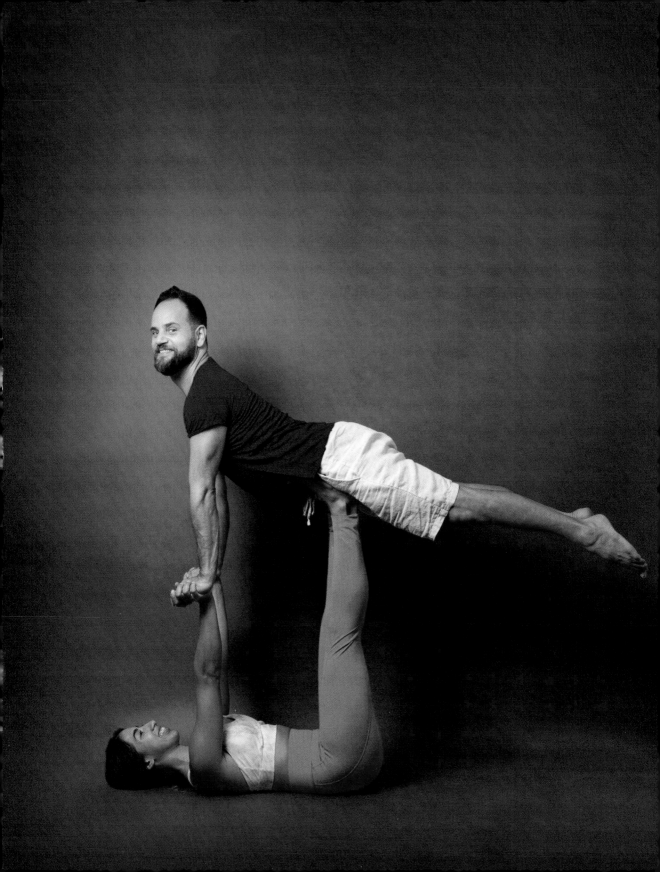

MOVE, CONNECT, PLAY

THE ART AND SCIENCE OF ACROYOGA

JASON NEMER

ST. MARTIN'S
ESSENTIALS
NEW YORK

First published in the United States by St. Martin's Essentials, an imprint of St. Martin's Publishing Group

MOVE, CONNECT, PLAY. Copyright © 2022 by Jason Nemer. All rights reserved. Printed in the United States of America. For information, address St. Martin's Publishing Group, 120 Broadway, New York, NY 10271.

www.stmartins.com

Designed by Steven Seighman and A. "Rising" McDowell

Cover photographs: Ramon Frias
Interior photographs: Aggelos Anastasiou, Erik Nemer, Julio Bajdaun, Justin Bench, Justin Caruso, Kadri Kurgan, Louis 'Fish' Fisher, Nouredeen Ahmed Saber
Models: Amy Salguero, Christine Falaguerra, Eddie Salguero Jr., Evangelia Mosiou, Eve Modens, John Karvelis, Jonathan Rea, Laura Labron, Melinda Thompson, Nouredeen Ahmed Saber, Polet Mehrabian, Reem Hamed Abdellatif, Sarah Solomon
Artwork: Eleni Hadjisavva

Library of Congress Cataloging-in-Publication Data

Names: Nemer, Jason, author.
Title: Move, Connect, Play : The Art and Science of AcroYoga / Jason Nemer.
Description: First edition. | New York : St. Martin's Essentials, 2021. | Includes index.
Identifiers: LCCN 2021002089 | ISBN 9781250774170 (trade paperback) |
    ISBN 9781250774187 (ebook)
Subjects: LCSH: Hatha yoga. | Acrobatics. | Exercise for couples.
Classification: LCC RA781.7 .N453 2021 | DDC 613.7/046—dc23
LC record available at https://lccn.loc.gov/2021002089

Our books may be purchased in bulk for promotional, educational, or business use. Please contact your local bookseller or the Macmillan Corporate and Premium Sales Department at 1–800-221-7945, extension 5442, or by email at MacmillanSpecialMarkets@macmillan.com.

First Edition: 2022

10 9 8 7 6 5 4 3 2 1

CONTENTS

PREFACE

HOW TO USE THIS BOOK

The practices shared in this book will not only change your life, they will also make you better at relating to others. I have had the unique privilege of witnessing thousands of people from all walks of life create profound connections by playing like children do and literally stacking themselves on top of one another in various shapes and forms. As a fun and dynamic way to move, connect, and play, AcroYoga has grown to reach over one hundred countries in just under twenty years.

As much as this book is a step-by-step guide to doing AcroYoga, it is also a guide to becoming the best version of yourself. From that place, you continue the journey by becoming the best partner you can be. This book is for every person at every skill level, and for anyone who wants to have more fun. Whether you're a beginner or an expert, the principles shared here are foundational and serve all people. I've designed the content to speak to the what, how, and why of AcroYoga and its three roots—acrobatics, therapeutics, and yoga. As you're reading I invite you to explore all the chapters and feel free to pick and choose your points of entry. At the end of most chapters you will find principles and practices to help you retain and really experience the uplifting power of AcroYoga for yourself, even if you don't have a partner yet.

As you read this book you will be empowered with more tools to strengthen your relationships and navigate the highs and lows of your life. You will become more fit, agile, and balanced. You will find more opportunities for fun, healing, and personal growth. And with millions of people already practicing AcroYoga, you will meet new and exciting friends from all over the world. If you're nodding your head yes, then this practice is for you!

If you're wondering if you can do this, I promise you can. I have spent much of my adult life listening to people insist they cannot do something, only to prove them wrong moments later. My secret? Small, progressive steps that give clear instruction on how you can safely and easily learn to say 'yes' to AcroYoga, 'yes' to the unknown, and 'yes' to living a happier, more fulfilling life.

A big source of our happiness and sadness stems from our feelings of being connected to or seperate from others. My intention is to invite you to become a part of the global AcroYoga community. What's in it for you is a lifetime of human connection, learning, playing and growing. For those of you who are one of the millions already practicing AcroYoga, the insights I share in this book will help you understand the foundation of your practice so you can get even more out of it. From there, your life will gain depth and take new turns you never could have expected.

When you learn a new system, you can be like a child filled with wonder and excitement. Every system you learn becomes another lens through which you can see the world. The lenses I'll explore with you in these pages include yoga, acrobatics, healing, physics, Taoism, Hinduism, Buddhism, neuroscience, and even chemistry. This kaleidoscope of perspectives will help you examine your life, relationships and beliefs, leading you

to find more clarity in how you want to invest your energy. When you start to see yourself and others through these new lenses, you will have opened the door to rewriting your worldview.

I write from my perspective as a street-trained sociologist guided by the lessons and principles of dozens of movement masters, healers, and yogis. I offer you my findings after thirty-three years of acrobatics training, eighteen years of AcroYoga training, and reaching national and world championships in partner acrobatics. I am compelled to share my perspective with the world in the hope that it helps make our home a better place—one where adults play more and we can relearn to build community based on real human experiences.

The foundations of AcroYoga will have you moving between acrobatics and therapeutics, helping you find balance and yoga along the way. You will know you're doing it "right" if you are having a good time and learning. You will gain obvious physical skills from this practice, like how to balance someone's full body weight on your feet. But you will also learn how the words you use influence your mental state, and how your thoughts affect every aspect of your life. AcroYoga has the power to change not only the body you are in, but also the direction your life is going. No matter which door you open first, you are stepping into a realm of possibilities that will undoubtedly expand what you think is possible for yourself.

The core content of *Move, Connect, Play* is organized by the AcroYoga Table of Elements—a singular source of information about the static poses that make up this movement language. This book is also full of stories that offer insight into how the practice can affect you on more profound levels. Reading this book will give you deep insight into the theories of AcroYoga. However, the magic of this practice is in the present-moment connections you share with people as you actually practice it. It all starts with your first flight. From there, your horizons for movement, connection and play will expand and you will become part of a beautiful international community that has already changed the world through the mutual support of AcroYoga.

MONKEY BUSINESS

If you ever played "airplane" as a kid then you already know about the energy that naturally flows between two humans doing AcroYoga. That energy is the seed from which has grown everything you will read about in this book. That energy is natural, it is fun, and it can become part of your life again. Looking back on where I started from where I am now, I would have thought you were crazy if you told me years ago that I would one day start a worldwide movement based on play. My story is one of big dreams, meeting the right people, dedicating myself to disciplines, and learning from masters. What I am about to share with you completely transformed my life and continues to change the lives of countless others.

With thousands of certified teachers in over seventy countries, AcroYoga is truly a global practice. But I didn't build this movement alone. There have been many collaborators throughout the years who helped spread this practice around the world. The first time I met AcroYoga's co-founder, Jenny Sauer-Klein, we stayed up until five in the morning playing, discussing, and dreaming of how we could combine our bags of tricks to make a new movement language that would be approachable to anyone. As accomplished acrobats who had already discovered the power of yoga and healing arts, we also saw a unique opportunity to create a practice that would allow people like us, with advanced training in one discipline, to enrich their lives by exploring complementary skill sets. The spark that was lit that evening with Jenny has allowed millions of people around the world to rediscover the joy and magic of human connection.

I believe that the elements of AcroYoga are part of our human DNA. From the favelas in Brazil to the rural rice fields in Thailand, and from the parks of London to the beaches of California, I've seen adults suspending children on their feet in the game of "airplane." These "games" are not unique to our species. Our closest relatives, Bonobo apes, exhibit many different trust games that include risk and fun. Their social structure, like ours, is supported by various types of interaction including play, grooming, and otherwise caring for friends and relatives.

For us human primates, AcroYoga is a social innovation that helps people of all ages, from all cultures, experience connection with one another in ways that are fun, meaningful, and encourage our growth. From the beginning, this practice was designed to reach all people: old and young, tall and short, fit and not so fit. As teachers and trailblazers of this new movement art, we have built a system and a community that emphasizes inclusivity, sustainability and balance. No matter your size, skill, or fitness level, there is always more to learn.

AcroYoga is both a solo journey that expands who you are as an individual, and a partner practice that plugs you into a community. These practices can reveal new levels of depth and understanding in who we really are. The good news and the bad news are the same: there is no end to what you will discover as you learn to base, fly, and spot your friends, family, and strangers (or what I like to call, "the

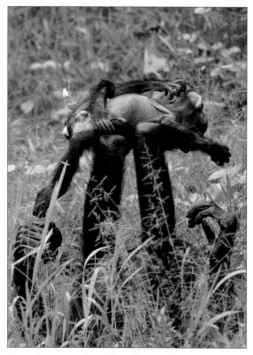

Bonobo apes bonding through trust games

friends you haven't flown yet"). As an individual, you'll learn to connect to your breath, your strengths, your obstacles, and your true self. As a partner you will learn to listen, communicate your needs, and build trust. In community you will learn to give and receive support in an exponentially scalable way. This inner growth naturally leads to us becoming pillars of strength in our relationships and the world.

Blending the three infinitely vast disciplines of acrobatics, yoga, and therapeutics has both benefits and challenges. One of the benefits is the discovery that at the heart of each practice are many common principles and universal truths. For example, as you learn how to align your bones with gravity, that will make your movement smarter, stronger, and more sustainable. The challenge comes in learning how to make something unique and better than the sum of its parts while still honoring the methods that have worked for centuries. I have tried many things throughout the years that did not pair well, were not sequenced well, or were just a hot mess! Once, I decided to give my Thai massage teacher's daughter an acrobatic performance after doing six hours of Thai massage. I was so relaxed

and chilled out that I ended up dropping my partner on the first move! Blending things takes practice to do well and often we learn the hard way how not to combine things. The blending became even more interesting as the practice of AcroYoga spread around the globe, and was expanded upon by many different types of people—from dancers and circus artists to traditional yogis, fitness buffs, and everyday people.

Because it is so multi-faceted, AcroYoga has the potential to touch so many aspects of wellness. Physically you will gain strength, flexibility, and improved balance. Mentally you will become more grounded, present, and clear. Emotionally you will develop more tools to feel, communicate, problem-solve, and exchange support. In any given AcroYoga experience, we have the potential to enter into deep states of meaningful connection as we take risks, build trust, and have fun with one another. These states of yoga, or union, can range from acrobatic to therapeutic, in the air to on the ground, from exhilaration to meditation.

At the ground level, AcroYoga is supported by my own life experience, my family, and my many teachers. To illustrate where AcroYoga came from, I'd like to share the story of how I gathered the skills, knowledge, and experiences that eventually became the heart of this global practice.

THE BEGINNINGS OF ACROYOGA

I was born in Mexico and raised in the United States with all the benefits and drawbacks of a mixed-heritage immigrant family. My mother and father were both second-generation citizens in their respective countries, the US and Mexico. During the late '60s, America was a land of change, opportunity, and uncertainty. There was a popular phrase at the time: "America—love it or leave it." And my mom, being the eighteen-year-old rebellious hippie she was, decided to leave it, married my dad, and set out on a ten-year adventure in Mexico and Venezuela not knowing a word of Spanish. She was my first teacher and is to this day one of my best friends. Some of the things she learned, and later taught me, were the power of learning another language, the beauty of steeping in different cultures, and the courage it takes to leave your home country. I had no idea these values would lead me on my own ten-year adventure around the world many years

later. It was all part of a divine plan I would one day see in retrospect. Learning to let go of home and to embrace being an outsider has helped me develop compassion for myself and for others feeling alone. It has helped me find ways to be welcomed and accepted in countless cultures across the globe.

My mom's father died when I was three. I have a few memories of him, but it wasn't until my grandmother passed away in my twenties that I discovered a

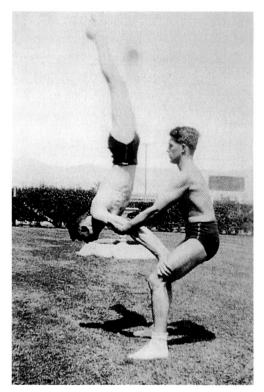

Jason's grandfather (left) doing partner acrobatics, circa 1940

family secret. Going through old photos with my mother, I came across snapshots of Grandpa doing real-deal partner acrobatics in Southern California in the 1940s. As it turned out, I had both nature and nurture working in my favor as I learned to interact with the world as an AcroYogi. At an early age, I was already very focused and fearless. My mom called me "the tank" because I would not crawl around things—I often crawled right over huge obstacles, headed right toward whatever I had my eyes on.

At five years old my parents divorced. As difficult as that transition was, I gained two stepparents who had a big influence on my life. My stepfather, John, was a marriage and family counselor who did hypnosis on his patients. He taught a treasure trove of communication and listening techniques, and his teachings greatly influenced how I learned to interact with others. From active listening and echoing to emotional responsibility, I was equipped from a young age with powerful tools for interconnection. I'll never forget when he told me, "Nobody can make you mad," a phrase that has stuck with me to this day. I learned that emotional responsibility is a choice, and that we can always choose how we relate to the situations we are faced with, rather than being subject to the first emotion that surfaces.

Apart from being born in Mexico and having a non-traditional family, I grew up in California with all the privileges that come with living there. My life took an exciting turn when I set my first big life goal at the tender age of nine. It was 1984 and I was watching the Summer Olympics, glued to the TV while my brothers and cousins played outside. In those few hours, I was sucked into a wild new dreamland where people had Jedi powers that enabled them to fly, flip, and do things I didn't know were possible. The US gymnastics team won gold that year. I remember deciding clearly, right then and there, that I wanted to go to that party someday. It was the first big dream I'd ever had and it was substantial enough to keep me chasing after it for over a decade.

Three years after watching the Olympics, I tagged along with my little brother to my first gymnastics class. I didn't stand out as particularly talented or built for the sport, but I had a great time and kept going back. By age thirteen, I had begun competing in men's gymnastics. In gymnastics it all starts and ends with your body and mind. There are no partners—it is you, six events, gravity, and skill. Of course, I was assisted (I believe nowadays the word would be "tormented") by a coach on the side who pushed me past many fears (and a lot of physical pain). I gained solo mastery of dynamic power, balance, strength, flexibility, rolling, bailing out, flipping, tumbling, swinging, jumping, unifying, competing, and the wisdom of progressive training. I would not be the acrobat I am today had I not started with traditional gymnastics. I am forever grateful for the courage and discipline I gained during those formative years.

Barely six months into my gymnastics career I caught my first glimpse of partner acrobatics. It was jaw-dropping, like falling in love for the first time. I saw a small girl do a handstand on a huge, sturdy man's hands, and I knew I had to meet these people. I went right up to them and asked if I could try. I flew my first candlestick shoulderstand and the rest is history.

In my first year competing in partner acrobatics, I was a thirteen-year-old base paired with a seven-year-old flyer, David. In those early years I competed in both gymnastics and partner acrobatics. While I was learning how to balance and throw my own body around with gymnastics, I was also learning how to balance and throw David around in acrobatics.

One of the things I learned early in my career was that fun is an essential component of training. I remember the first gymnastics magazine I ever bought. It featured a Russian gymnast standing on the first-place podium without even a hint of joy. In second place was a Chinese gymnast with not one happy muscle flexed in any part of her face. Finally, the bronze medalist was an American who was beaming from ear to ear. I wanted to be the best, but I also wanted to enjoy the process. I would train hard—but not in a negative environment.

My gymnastics coach at the time did not offer the type of training environment I wanted. He was physically abusive and overly demanding. He walked around the gym with a stick he called the "Straight Leg Indicator." We would be struck by the stick if our legs were not straight or toes not pointed, which amounted to many times per training session. We were only shown kindness on the rare occasions that we tried a very difficult skill or demonstrated perfect form. Within a few short years of gymnastics training, it became clear that my Olympic dream as a gymnast was not realistic, and the cross-training of gymnastics and partner acrobatics ended when I was fifteen. I was ready to pour my entire heart into becoming the best acrobat in the world.

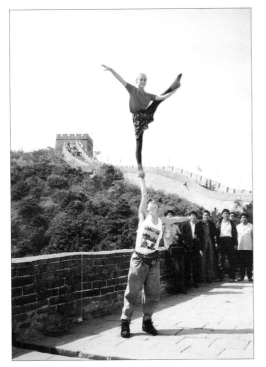

Jason at age 16 in China for the Jr. World Championships in Sports Acrobatics

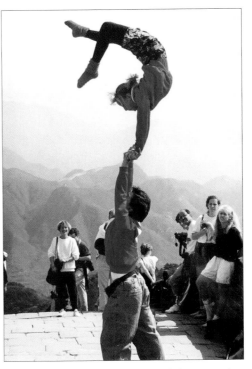

Jason basing flyer Amber Malchow on the Great Wall of China, 1991

Just one year later, at sixteen, I got close. I won a silver medal and two bronze medals at the Jr. World Championships in Sports Acrobatics held in Beijing in 1991. By age nineteen I had become one of America's best acrobats and coaches, winning both Coach of the Year and Athlete of the Year in 1994 at the USA National Championships for Sports Acrobatics. That same year, I designed and submitted the developmental training program for competitive American

acrobats that is still in use today. I was firing on all cylinders as a world-class acrobat, and I was clear on my next goal: win the Senior World Cup and one day represent the United States as an acrobat in the Olympic Games. Unfortunately, sports acrobatics was not and is still not an Olympic sport. Even so, I was still able to reach my life goal of being in the Olympics when I was invited to perform in the 1996 Summer Olympics Opening Ceremonies in Atlanta, Georgia. In that twelve-year journey from seeing the Games on TV to taking part in person, I learned to be driven in reaching my dreams yet flexible in how I got there.

Unlike acrobatics, yoga came to me in many little waves over the years, beginning with my mom who taught me how to do shoulderstands during TV commercials and took me to get my transcendental meditation mantra when I was four. While I didn't know it then, all my gymnastics warm-ups were filled with yoga poses. By the time I took my first proper yoga class in college, I'd already had ten years of practice in things like splits, wheels, and straddles. Nevertheless, that class blew my mind and catalyzed huge changes in my life. By the time I graduated from University of California, San Diego in 2001, I was spiritually activated and ready for much more yoga.

My grandmother passed away that year, leaving me with an inheritance that bought me time to explore this new side of myself and not rush into a career decision. That time was like a rite of passage: I was reading five spiritual books at once, became fully vegetarian, and started looking into yoga teacher trainings. I completed my first yoga teacher training in the summer of 2003, and after receiving my certification I moved to San Francisco, the then-epicenter of America's rapidly growing yoga culture.

By twenty-eight years old, I was armed with a degree in economics, a yoga teaching certification, and a job teaching trampoline and acrobatics at one of the top circus training centers in the US. But I had little savings, and whatever money I made would go toward my next meal or my next yoga class. I considered getting a restaurant job, but after making a resume and preparing to go job-hunting, a strong voice inside of me told me to put the resume down and reconsider. Deep down I knew that yoga was so much more than a ninety-minute class to me—it was an all-encompassing philosophy quickly affecting all parts of my life. I decided to fully commit to making a living based on my passions.

Then I met Jenny, AcroYoga's co-founder, on December 20, 2003. We had heard about each other many times through mutual friends, and our meeting was super magical. I held her in my hands in that same handstand I had seen back when I was twelve. She therapeutically flew me, or in other words, she balanced me upside down on her feet as I breathed, relaxed, and was stretched in the most delicious way. We did not know what we had just unlocked, but we knew it was something big.

Jenny had trained with Nateshvar Ken Scott, the creator of Contact Yoga, in which therapeutic flying has its origins. His students, Kevin and Erin O'Keefe, went on to found Circus Yoga, a discipline designed to share circus arts with families. From these three teachers, Jenny learned many things that became some of the most potent seeds for AcroYoga. Jenny also taught circus arts to children, so she had many beginner-friendly ways to teach acrobatics to civilians. She brought a complementary softness and receptivity to my fire and focus on progressive systems. At our "office"—Dolores Park in San Francisco—we spent years jamming, teaching, and expanding what AcroYoga was. Together we developed a holistic system based on what we found by practicing, playing, and exploring all the ways our bodies could acrobatically synchronize. Our partnership was the catalyst that created the practice of AcroYoga. After a few years of developing content, we decided to make an instructional book for our students. Halfway through drafting the book we wondered, *Maybe we should teach people how to teach this stuff* . . .

So a few years later, in 2006, we led our first AcroYoga Teacher training. The seventeen students who came were proof that we could make a living doing what we loved. Not only could we change people's lives through this practice, but they could help us scale the whole thing by learning to unlock the potential of yet more students. We went from that first training at a friend's vineyard in the Santa Cruz mountains to the dusty *playa* of Black Rock City for AcroYoga's debut at the infamous Burning Man festival. Back in 2006, nobody really knew what AcroYoga was, but there were hundreds of people doing contact improv dance at Center Camp, the main gathering place for the festival. Of the seventeen graduates from that first teacher training, about half of them came to Burning Man to test their skills and teach humans to fly.

One of the most notable new AcroYogis I got on my feet was Sergey Brin, the co-founder of Google. To me, at the time I flew him he was just another flyer, but he was instantly hooked and became a regular student of the art of basing and flying. The next year I was invited to share AcroYoga at his 32nd birthday party. His home was modest (for a billionaire), and he treated me like family as we ate barbecued chicken and corn on the cob off of paper plates on his balcony. He went on to attend some festivals that I organized, and when he came to a five-day AcroYoga immersion I taught in New York City, he invited me to his place there where he gave me one of the best compliments of my career: We were reflecting on what he had learned at the immersion when he said, "I am very impressed with the culture you have created with AcroYoga." Coming from the man who created one of the biggest companies in the world, including the Google campus and countless innovations for team and system building, it gave

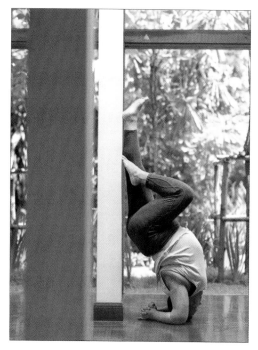

AcroYoga is for all people: Golff Dudjid of Body Positive Thailand Yoga

me a moment of pause. I knew I was a skilled acrobat and teacher, but I was beginning to see that the power of what I was creating lay in the practice's approach to human relationships. Many things have changed from those early days of AcroYoga, but many will always be the same. What has changed are the levels, styles, and complexity of the practice; what has stayed the same is how people interact and grow in AcroYoga environments.

As I began traveling to teach AcroYoga, I noticed that people loved watching it, but there was a disconnect between what they believed they could do and what they were truly capable of. In 2017 at a yoga retreat in Thailand, I met an amazing yogini named Golff Dudjid. She is a pioneer of Body Positive Thailand Yoga, a practice focused on accepting your body as is and building a positive relationship with it. Being a large woman, she would not let me fly her in the beginning, but she kept a watchful eye from a safe distance as I flew everyone else at the retreat, including large men. Finally after many invitations she said yes. Fears, insecurities, and other unwanted emotions are like logs: they contain years of stored energy and when the right conditions present themselves, this potential energy transforms to kinetic energy. How this manifested for Golff was a two-minute flight where she was giggling, laughing, and screaming, "Jason, don't drop me, Jason, oh my God!" Everyone around us could not help but smile and giggle too. We all saw and felt the stored energy that Golff had accumulated for years finally bursting into flames as she leaned into me and trusted that she was in a safe place to convert fear into joy.

I share these stories to show you that AcroYoga is designed to be accessible to all people. Just recently, that design faced its biggest test. In 2018, thousands of people from Honduras, Guatemala, and other Latin American countries were fleeing dangerous conditions in their homelands by walking thousands of miles toward the US–Mexico border. Upon arrival, they were met with a harsh and unwelcoming border wall fortified by the Trump administration's policy on immigration. The day before Thanksgiving in 2018, I was invited to this political and humanitarian hot spot by Vandana Hart, the creator of the Netflix series *We Speak Dance*. Vandana got together a group of ten movers and shakers to go to the border in Tijuana to welcome and perform for the caravan of refugees coming to seek asylum in America.

Crossing the border into Mexico from the US could not have been easier for us,

but getting into the border camp took hours. We just wanted to get in, play some music, dance, and share AcroYoga. After a lot of sweet talking we were finally given permission to enter. The people and the place were not clean by any standard, but as soon as we got past the gate I lay down on my back and flew some children on my feet. Their giggles were contagious. It instantly lightened the mood to see unfiltered, unscripted joy in a dark situation. As the fun spread, even a few adults joined in on the party! There was so much laughter. Vandana and her dance crew started busting moves and the tired, drained refugees who had literally walked thousands of miles began to dance too. The party grew so large that we were escorted to a nearby football field to make space for more.

For more than an hour, we celebrated life through movement and connection. None of these people had ever done AcroYoga, but everyone wanted to trust, play, and connect in spite of their conditions being unimaginably poor. US border officers had been granted permission to use lethal force if there was a rush on the border, and just an hour after we left the camp there was a shooting. With all those negative conditions in context, sharing AcroYoga at the refugee camp was one of the most meaningful exchanges I have ever had. To be able to bring hope and smiles to people who had nothing, and to see people who were afraid to trust let their guard down, was life changing for everyone there. What moved me were the deep bonds of friendship these people had cultivated during their dangerous journey. They left their homelands and all their possessions behind to embark on this new chapter of their lives.

The next day, Thanksgiving, I drove north to Sacramento to be with my family. I pulled into a coffee shop to get a snack for the drive and while standing in line, I witnessed so much suffering in the people around me. Everyone was on their phones and there was a thick layer of disconnection and tension in the air due to holiday stress and obligations. These people had so much more in life, yet they lacked the simple joys the refugees had. By sharing AcroYoga at the border camp, I had not only lifted the refugees up, they had also lifted me to see how strong, beautiful, and valuable true human connection is, and that AcroYoga has the power to connect in spite of cultural differences.

2018 was a big year for expanding who I shared the practice with. On top of bringing AcroYoga to the border camp,

I also had the pleasure and honor of flying three paraplegic friends that year. (I had thousands of flights under my belt before taking on the risk of flying people with debilitating injuries.) The first was a childhood acrobat friend who had suffered a bike accident that left her paralyzed. She had metal rods along her spine and I did not know what to expect as I got her into the air, but it was a great success and she giggled the whole time! The second was a Lebanese AcroYogi who was shot by an Israeli soldier in the occupied lands of Palestine. He was shocked by what we were able to do. Within just a few breaths we were able to bring new space to his entire spine. The third paraplegic I flew that year was Leon Ford. He was presenting at an event I attended in Los Angeles called Summit Series. He caught my eye at the presenters' dinner because he came in with his wheelchair. Toward the end of the night I made my way over to talk to him and said, "Hi, my name is Jason and I want to invite you to do something that will blow your mind. I want to fly you." He really had no idea what I was talking about, but he looked up at me with his big brown eyes and a huge smile and said, "Who would say no to that?" We left the dinner and had about a ten-minute walk back to the

Summit venue. I offered to push him but he said, "I like building strength so I rarely have people push me." He was not born disabled, but was the victim of police brutality: At a traffic stop in Pittsburgh, Pennsylvania, he was pulled over by an officer and shot five times. He survived but lost the use of half his body. After hearing about his spiritual awakening inspired by his experience, and feeling the light and positivity behind his words and actions, I was so excited to fly him! Sure enough we had an amazing time. Even better, when he came down, he decided to base people on his hands. He did not see or feel limitations; he felt free, supported, and connected. Now when people say they can't do AcroYoga, I have three real-life stories of people who said 'yes' in spite of their obstacles. We just have to find the right ways to play.

What I have experienced over the past few decades has helped me crack the code of what makes us click in relation to one another. People are blown away by what is possible when they connect and exchange the oldest human currency—trust. AcroYoga has universal appeal because we all have the same human desires: we long for connection, support, and fun. This social experiment of building AcroYoga has broken through many cultural and mental

barriers over the years and has given me faith that our human spirits are far more similar than they are different. No matter what language you speak, AcroYoga is a common code that dissolves other barriers to communication. Now, after many years dedicating myself to conducting experiments and testing my theories, AcroYoga has a stable foundation—one that has been designed to empower all people.

ONE BILLION STRONG

We support all people through movement, connection, and play.
—ACROYOGA MISSION STATEMENT

Back in 2016, I was in an airport lounge with AcroYoga's then CEO, Rahel Ben-Cnaan, brainstorming a rebranding of AcroYoga. We were discussing changing the logo and colors, and clarifying the mission statement when she asked me, "What is Jason Nemer's life mission?" When I thought about it, it had to do with empowering people to believe in themselves and to trust others. On a napkin we scribbled out this mission and it has been a guiding light ever since.

I believe the world is already a better place with the millions of AcroYogis playing in parks, at home, at work, and anywhere there is space to lie down and lift people up. This book is full of the priceless life lessons and training techniques that many masters have taught me in the last thirty years, and in reading it you will learn how to use these principles to turn joy, empowerment, and trust into lasting parts of your life.

From one peak we can see others and create new goals and missions. What I realized a few years back is that the mission of AcroYoga can help us reach a new milestone: In my lifetime I aim to see one billion AcroYoga practitioners sharing the joys of embodied play. This idea was planted as I stood on the Olympic stage in 1996. The Opening Ceremonies of the Olympic Games are one of the most widely watched events in the world. What I felt in that stadium when I saw sixty thousand faces looking back at me was a sense of the whole world coming together. Those faces could not have been more diverse—so many colors of skin, clothing, flags, and different gestures—yet what

united them was their desire to see all the world's best athletes come together. And while only some people get to attend the Olympics, we all deserve to feel that sense of global unity.

Once two people know how to do basic AcroYoga, they no longer need a common verbal language. A Tibetan flyer, a Colombian base, and a Norwegian spotter can grow a friendship based on trust, respect, and fun; smiles and high-fives are universally understood and appreciated. Once there are a billion AcroYogis, I believe the world will be forever changed by our collective ability to drop in on an essential level with anyone, anywhere. Our ability to unlock our genetic potential is directly linked to our capacity to lean into one another. As of November 2021, there are over 3 million posts on Instagram with the hashtag #AcroYoga. Through AcroYoga I believe we can reach incredible levels of individual and collective potential, and this book is a roadmap for that dream: to unify the world through movement, connection, and play.

PART I
THE FOUNDATION

THE METHOD

Movement, Connection, and Play

In my life as an acrobat and movement teacher, I have spent thousands of hours observing the physical shapes and complex movement patterns of the human body. Regardless of the style or discipline, I have found that the foundational qualities and concepts of human movement are the same around the world because we are all governed by the same physical laws.

Over time I have used the scientific method to organize my observations, and through that process I have been able to distill my insights about human movement and connection into the key practices and principles that are featured in this book. After decades of teaching movement to children and adults in dozens of countries, I can say with confidence that the magic ingredients that turn people's lives upside down can be boiled down to movement, connection, and play. In the next several pages, I will share what it is about this combination

that is so powerful and essential for humans to live a full and happy life.

This planet has seen a huge variety of life-forms over the past 3.5 billion years. From single-celled organisms floating in the primordial sea to billions of humans climbing to the top of the food chain with unprecedented dominance, life has evolved a lot. I enjoy looking at life at its extremes—from the big to the small, the seen to the unseen. Human beings have evolved into one of the most unique and complex expressions of life in the known universe. Our bodies have organs that are made of tissues, that are made of cells, that are made of compounds, that are made of atoms, that are made of space, energy, and matter. From the obvious to the subtle, we are thoughts, words, actions, feelings, energy, vibration, and spirit. When analyzing the human experience, it is helpful to understand the many individual layers that make up the whole. When life is lived well these individual parts can be harmonized to maximize our happiness, wholeness, and oneness. If that sounds like a tall order, that's because it is, but you have your whole life to get better at it, and this book will offer you many different avenues to explore on your way there.

MOVEMENT

Nothing happens until something moves.
—ALBERT EINSTEIN

Movement is a natural expression of life. Each day water flows in its natural cycle from one place to another: giant icebergs melt into cold arctic oceans; sunshine evaporates the water back into clouds that rain; mighty rivers bring these water molecules back to the sea where they started their journey. Movement and temperature are different words for the same thing—a way to quantify energy. Take the example of water: At zero degrees Celcius water freezes, and at one hundred degrees it boils. There is an even more extreme temperature discovered by the scientist Lord Kelvin, who developed the Kelvin scale: He calculated a number called absolute zero. At this temperature

there is no molecular movement. Absolute zero defines one of the endpoints of movement. At each degree from absolute zero to a sunny beach day, molecules vibrate more and move faster until they reach a range where life and movement coexist. This sweet spot as we know it is roughly between minus 20 degrees and 120 degrees Celsius. Within this range of temperatures, life has the possibility to express and move as it has been doing on Earth for 3.5 billion years.

Movement defines life, and life evolves and adapts to its environments and unique situations. It is therefore important to know how we evolved to understand the movements for which we were designed. For thousands of years, Homo sapiens wandered the world in search of food and shelter like many other animals. We were not top predators until very recently; we were actually preyed upon by many other animals that had bigger muscles, teeth, and claws. However, we did develop an upright posture to see danger or food from farther away. We also developed huge brains and opposable thumbs that, over time, proved to offer us opportunities that other animals had not yet exploited.

As a species we evolved over three million years ago from a common ancestor called Australopithecus Afarensis. Lucy, as she is known, is the world's most famous early human. She had both ape and human features, including long ape-like arms and an upright posture. She stood about three and a half feet tall with a brain size similar to a modern chimpanzee. How we evolved as a species was based on our environmental pressures and opportunities: by taking advantage of those opportunities we were able to thrive and propagate. We had great diversity in how and where we moved based on the food sources we subsisted on. How we moved ranged from walking, running, and jumping to climbing, swinging, and swimming. Where we moved was all over God's green and icy earth! Early humans had active lifestyles that supported our health on many levels. We moved constantly to find wild food sources and avoid being eaten ourselves.

Our bodies communicate through movement and touch, and ultimately our senses are more at the core of how we learn about life and the world around us than things like spelling and long division. For the first year of human life there is little to no speech but there are thousands of hours of touch and millions of little movement breakthroughs that eventually culminate in our first steps.

On the macro level, life aligns with the movement and cycles of the sun and moon. The sun's cycles have directed our circadian rhythm since life began eons ago: Exposure to the sun in the morning tells our brains to produce serotonin, helping us be awake, focused, and happy. As the sun sets, our body temperature lowers and we get a dose of melatonin to help us get ready for dreamland. The moon affects the tides, our emotions, and women's menstrual cycles. From sunrise to sunset, new moon to full moon, crawling to running, and birth to death, movement is an essential aspect of life.

As complex as the human body is, there are a finite number of bones and angles that those bones are able to achieve. These parameters create the potential for human movement, and this potential can be put on a scale and measured. There are three primary factors that comprise your movement potential: strength, flexibility, and technique. They are the key ingredients that form any movement art. This is explained in more detail in later chapters, but for now they are important factors to know.

Human strength can be compared to the amount of horsepower in a car engine. You can have a powerful engine with exceptionally high horsepower, but if the car is extremely heavy the extra horsepower won't make you very fast. (Picture Shaquille O'Neal, for example.) On the other hand, you might have a smaller engine with less horsepower, but with an aluminum-frame car you can have a tremendous amount of speed (Bruce Lee, for example) because the car is lightweight. This concept is known as a strength-to-weight ratio.

Flexibility would be the car's turning radius, or how many degrees the wheels can rotate to make a sharp turn. Imagine your joints as the wheels.

Finally, technique is the art of maneuvering the car through a course without damaging it, using the right amount of power and acceleration. In our bodies, technique is the intelligence to operate the machines we are in. The human body may not be the best at any one thing—swinging, swimming, running, or climbing—but what is amazing about our vehicle is that with very little training we can do a bit of everything.

The coordination of our movement can be attributed to our cerebellum. This movement command center is located behind the top of the brain stem, where the spinal cord meets the brain. It receives information from our sensory organs, spinal cord, and other parts of the brain, then regulates our motor movements. It coordinates our posture, balance, and speech, resulting in smooth and coordinated muscular activity. Although it is a relatively small portion of the brain (about 10 percent by weight), it contains roughly half of the brain's neurons. We are built to move *from* our brains *to* our bodies—this is how we have evolved, and this is the genetic potential we can claim in our lives.

Our design as humans is a recent expression within the animal kingdom and an experimental design at best. The technical term for our most common form of movement is *bipedal locomotion*. This means our two feet are our main engines for movement. This frees our arms and hands to use tools, high-five our friends, pick fruit, and make housing structures. Our vertical design combined with our heavy heads puts a significant load on our spines. Everything in life has a cost and a benefit, and many of us pay for our upright stance and big brains with stiff backs and sore necks.

Our primate cousins rely on their arms to do more of the heavy lifting to get from point A to point B. They evolved a form of movement called *brachiation,* meaning their arms are their main engines for movement. This is a fancy way to say that they swing through the trees! Even though we have evolved away from this as our primary movement modality, we still have the joints and genetic memory to swing from the branches, Tarzan style.

Many other animals get by just fine as *quadrupeds*, meaning their four feet are their main engines for movement. The creatures with this design experience way less lower back pain than we do, but without the same ability to chuck a spear.

Our development of opposable thumbs gave us the ability to make many different tools. In the beginning, early man did not make anything too fancy. We were opportunistic omnivores on a good day, scavengers on a bad one. After a top predator would abandon a kill, we would sneak in and break the bones open with our tools to eat the marrow. The might of our intellect supported us to survive and succeed as a species, but we were far from the most dominant animal on earth. We followed other animals as a source of food and clothing, becoming wanderers and dreamers. Our nomadic

lives led us to become generalists: We are proficient at many things, not especially great at any one thing. We move faster than a sloth, but nothing compared to a cheetah. We can out-swim the cheetah, but dolphins would be highly amused by our flailing about in the sea. We can out-climb a dog, but our primate cousins would poke fun at our attempts to maneuver through the jungle canopy. Our adaptation toward generalism has engineered our bodies to get by doing many types of movement.

For there to be movement there has to be force, and where there is force there is energy. The law of conservation of energy states that energy can neither be created nor destroyed; rather, it can only be transformed or transferred from one form to another. For instance, chemical energy is converted to kinetic energy when a stick of dynamite explodes from its potential energy form. Much of what we do in AcroYoga and in life is dance with potential and kinetic energy—from static to dynamic, from inhale to exhale. Let's explore the laws of this energy together.

NEWTON'S LAWS OF MOTION

Sir Isaac Newton, one of the most influential physicists of all time, discovered many natural laws that govern motion. You can think of these laws like the rules of a game. The game is how we move our bodies through life.

First Law: Law of Inertia

An object either remains at rest or continues to move at a constant velocity unless acted upon by a force.

This law speaks to the concept of inertia. Inertia is usually discussed with regard to inanimate objects, but it can be applied to humans, too. In AcroYoga there are many static poses and eventually students learn how to transition from one pose to another. This first law teaches us how we control leaning into points of contact to become still and stable, or to co-create movement.

Second Law: F = ma

The force (F) of an object is equal to the mass (m) of that object multiplied by the acceleration (a) of the object.

This second law is one of the most vital to understanding how partners are moved. These variables dictate the amount of force needed to create movement. Acceleration is a change in velocity, and the greater it is, the greater the force of an object will be. The faster you can do push-ups, the more force you will have to lift your partners in AcroYoga. This is why moving quickly is an important part of martial arts and acrobatics. Speed is one of the essential spices in the movement palette of acrobats.

Third Law: Action-Reaction

When one body exerts a force on a second body, the second body simultaneously exerts a force equal in magnitude and opposite in direction on the first body.

The third law is related to how we interact with the earth and others' bodies in acrobatics, therapeutics, and yoga. For example, when attempting a handstand, as I push my arms and hands into the floor, the floor exerts an equal and opposite force that travels through my body, helping my body stay inverted over my hands. This is how and why bone alignment with the earth and with one another is vital to finding ease in AcroYoga.

THE CURSE OF MODERN SEDENTARY LIFE

Long before Newton's time humans knew how to move as it was vital to their survival. Survive we did; thrive and spread around the globe we did too. Around ten thousand years ago humans started a revolution that has affected our health and happiness more than anything (possibly with the exception of smartphones). We began the drastic shift from being hunters and gatherers to being farmers. We learned how to domesticate animals and plants. (Or maybe more accurately, plants and animals began to domesticate us!) Settling down in one geographic area offered us new comforts and opportunities. With farming and raising livestock, our food sources became more abundant and predictable. However, the dense concentration of animals and humans in small spaces made us susceptible to contracting new viruses and illnesses that were never seen in our nomadic past. For all the benefits of having your next meal readily available, there are just as many if not more substantial and unpredictable costs.

The COVID-19 pandemic of 2020 is the most recent major expression of this modern reality. We've taken more and more steps away from our original ways of living; today there are very few humans living as we did in the past. Anthropologists have studied the lives and lifestyles of early hunter-gatherer societies, and the findings stand in stark contrast to the quality of life (or lack thereof) that we have rushed into at the speed of modernization. Consider this excerpt from Captain James Cook's journal entry about the native Maoris of New Zealand in 1772:

> *"As there is perhaps no source of disease either critical or chronic, but intemperance and inactivity, it cannot be thought strange that these people enjoy perfect and uninterrupted health: in all our visits to their towns, where young and old, men and women, crowded about us, prompted by the same curiosity that carried us to look at them, we never saw a single person who appeared to have any bodily complaint . . . a further proof that human nature is here untainted with disease, is the great number of old men that we saw, many of whom, by the loss of their hair and teeth, appeared to be very ancient, yet none of them were decrepit, and though not equal to the young in muscular*

strength, were not a whit behind them in cheerfulness and vivacity."

For many of our new technological advances we end up paying a heavy price, oftentimes unknowingly. We went from lives full of movement to lives full of sitting, typing, commuting, and slowly killing the wild parts of us that have been genetically cultivated over millions of years. We have become a domesticated, depressed version of our wild, true selves. Our literal and metaphorical cars have been upgraded with lots of technology, power windows, satellite radios, and so on, but they have lost peak performance on most levels—and they break down much more frequently.

As I write this, more than one billion adults, or 1 in 8 people across the globe, are overweight, and about a third of those adults are clinically obese. These numbers are the cumulative effects of our modern lifestyles. Things have gotten so easy for us that we hardly break a sweat unless we decide to in our artificial jungles—the gym. When we are done with our workouts we walk back to the car, and as luck would have it we got a great parking spot so we didn't need to walk far. On the ride home, we can drive through any number of places that will

give us a 2,000-calorie meal for under $10. By the end of the day, we go to sleep with a caloric surplus that is unnatural and unsustainable for us and the planet. In 2009, rates of obesity in the UK reached nearly a quarter of all the nation's adults—a fourfold increase in just thirty years. It has become such a concern that the National Health Secretary described childhood obesity as a "national emergency."

Modern life has changed the movement-loving primate into a caged version of its original self. In a recent study of six thousand adults in the US, 25 percent reported sitting for more than eight hours per day and 45 percent were inactive with little to no exercise all day. Only 3 percent of adults in the study reported sitting for less than four hours per day and being sufficiently active. My guess is they were professional athletes or AcroYogis.

FROM JUNGLES TO GYMS

My love-hate relationship with treadmills is ongoing, but if I had to choose between running on a treadmill or no movement at all, the choice would be easy—I'm running! Any movement is better than none. But, if faced with the choice of running on the treadmill or running outside, I would choose to go outdoors because being in nature offers many more benefits than running in a static indoor environment. Running outside forces you to be alert. What happens if there is a rock on the path? Or even better, what if there's a snake on the trail, or any of the countless things we cannot predict? A wild environment demands that our minds be present and alert.

Weightlifting can be another great way to move and increase your strength, but each movement practice comes with its benefits and drawbacks. In weightlifting, the drawbacks are that repeated motions with heavy weights can cause repetitive stress injuries over time. Also, many things we do in the gym are seated—a position we already overdo on average. For me, most exercises in the gym are a bit boring and soul-numbing. The benefits are tangible, but what if I could still get the post-workout glow by doing exercises that were super exciting instead? This is one of the many winning combos of AcroYoga.

I still love bench pressing—it's a go-to for many who work out in gyms. But a way to make it even more rewarding is to bench press a human on your hands! It is much more interesting and requires the complexity of using many stabilizing muscles that are easily missed in most workouts. When your weight giggles and encourages you to do two more reps, there is a decided advantage over lifting dumbbells. We have evolved to work with the chaos of the natural world by adapting and eventually harnessing it; but as a byproduct of our desire to control, gyms have taken us out of our natural movement environment. We can reclaim our old human potential when we move like the wild creatures we once were. It is more fun, too, so once you start you will find a natural motivation to keep pursuing this multidimensional way of playing in your body.

Using the treadmill versus running outside is like doing yoga for a workout versus developing an overall yogic awareness in your life. The physical practice alone is beneficial, but the benefits grow exponentially when you practice all the other aspects together (like non-attachment, mindfulness, meditation, breath control, etc.) You can get more out of your daily movements as you define what your goals are and expand the ways you challenge and support your body's movement potential.

THE MOVEMENT MIRACLE

If I could choose one remedy for humanity that would have the biggest impact on health and happiness, it would be functional movement. From the moment we are conceived, we grow, pulsate, and move for our whole lives. Many of the most important systems in our bodies function at their best when they are stimulated by movement. Obesity rates, depression, and many other conditions would be greatly reduced by daily doses of activity. Step one is realizing and deciding that movement can be part of our daily lives. From there, we can begin to make simple, impactful changes.

Do you have an elevator where you work? If so, you could take the stairs a few times per week, especially when you are mentally or emotionally off, to get into your body and press the reset button. Could you ride a bike to get your groceries? This has two benefits: first, you are moving, and second, you cannot buy as many things since you have to bring them back on a bike! As you find more daily movements you enjoy, you will unlock a new quality of life.

CONNECTION

You are related to everything alive. You share a common ancestor not just with all other human beings, but with your pets, and even the trees outside your window. Go back far enough and all our grandest of parents were the same cells in the ocean. Stand in the forest and all around you, from the towering trees to the ants crawling underneath your feet, are members of your extended family. Every second you are inhaling oxygen that flows into your blood and keeps your heart pumping. . . . When you eat other life, be it plants or animals, that life is transformed into the very composites that are your flesh and bones. You are not separate from mother nature. You are a part of it, from the air you breathe to the minerals in your toenails.

—JEVAN PRADAS

We were born because of the brave, sexy steps that our parents took toward each other. Being that we are mammals, we are connected to our mother's milk and kindness from birth. For many of us, our mother or father or both were there for us—feeding, cleaning, and holding us. As infants we have no concept of self; we just exist in a body—growing, learning, playing, and connecting to our internal world and the world around us. Around eighteen months into life we begin to recognize ourselves in the mirror. This illusion of individuality and separation grows and persists throughout our lives.

There are many plants and animals that are more deeply rooted in the awareness of community than self-identity and ego. Aspen trees often share a single root structure within the same aspen grove, so what appears as one individual tree is actually just part of a bigger underground organism. The way that fish school, birds flock, and ants colonize is an expression of unity, connection, and the natural order of how much of life organizes. As much as we need protein, sugars, and fats, we also crave the deep nourishment of human connection. From these first relationships between infants and caregivers we inevitably expand into our first friendships and become part of our first communities. We have our first fights over our toys being taken from us. We feel fear and loneliness and many of the human emotions that make connection such a key component of our emotional wellness.

As we grow older we learn more about who we are and how our self-knowledge relates to others. Am I a person who likes a lot of space and personal time, or do I crave closeness and intimacy? Where do these desires and potential imbalances come from? In what ways can I solicit my friends and community to support me as I learn who I am and what I need to be fulfilled in life? How can I provide the same gifts to others? We can create and co-create the life we want, and support others to do the same, by engaging with practices that connect us. Without these vital threads we can become depressed, lose our sense of purpose, and suffer many physical effects.

But with all of this philosophy of connection, there is an ironic twist: On a subatomic level, we never actually "touch" anything. We are made up of mostly empty space with little bits of matter and energy flying around at blistering speeds in very small circles. By definition, an electron will never touch another electron as they both are negatively charged. And because electrons are what are on the periphery of every surface we come into contact with, nothing can truly touch anything else. You're probably thinking, *But what do you mean, I know I touch my fork when I eat, right?* Not really, but it's easy to think that. Our brains do the best they can to understand our surroundings. The world seems flat and the sun revolves around the earth, right? Science has given us new lenses through which we can understand what is happening that we cannot see directly.

On the other hand, our emotional system does not care about what the electrons do. We have evolved to need touch and human closeness. Not all members of the animal kingdom are built with this thirst for connection: Black widow spiders earned their name for their brutal mating practice that ends poorly for most male spiders. In the bizarre post-coital ritual, the inseminated female murders her lover and eats him! Genes dictate many of our actions and interactions with the world around us; many animals live most of their lives in solitude with very brief moments to exchange genetic information before returning to solitude. But mammals have evolved to desire and be supported by some amount of connection.

The word connection comes from the Latin *conectare,* meaning "to join together." Basically, it's another word for *yoga*, or the ability to be in a state of unity. Connection can be defined in relation to yourself, other humans, or ultimately to everything that exists. We are all linked through our environment, and no matter how individual you may feel, your roots lie in the same earth as those of all other humans. Our survival as a species demands that we develop and invest in interpersonal relationships.

Connection covers a wide spectrum of human experiences, but it all starts with ourselves as we connect to the vehicles into which we were born. The human body is vast! It is made up of around 15 trillion cells that make up 206 bones, around six hundred muscles, and seventy-eight organs. There are tendons, ligaments, and other soft tissues holding this moving work of art together. With all of these variable tissues, one could go into a cave and never run out of human movement experiments. Many yogis, sages, and seekers did just that to learn about the body-mind-spirit triad and how these layers relate to each other, and many of their discoveries and insights are featured in this book.

Some animals at birth can run, jump, swim, and even hunt. Their advantage is clear and simple: Those babies are less vulnerable and adapt more quickly to supporting themselves. The animals born ready for independent life have little need for social skills. Humans, on the other hand, need more intensive care at birth and take longer to develop; as a result we gain a more comprehensive emotional and social structure. This adaptation has led to other evolutionary advantages such as teamwork, food sharing, and the ability to empathize and feel compassion. Our design dictates our actions to a large degree, and ideally our actions match our design to optimize health.

It took over two hundred thousand years of human history for the world's population to reach one billion, and only two hundred years more to reach seven billion. With all these people surely nobody is ever lonely or lacking in human connection, right? The question becomes one of quality versus quantity of interaction. In prehistoric tribes people were deep in connection because their lives depended on it; for countless generations we lived in nomadic bands of thirty to seventy humans because it was the sweet spot for food sharing and decision-making. Imagine if there were one thousand humans in a tribe in Africa thousands of years ago deciding where to go for their next meal. This large size would be inefficient and in hard times

people would die due to lack of cohesion. Humans evolved to live in smaller groups of immediate family, cousins, aunts and uncles, and of course elders. Trust was a real currency that increased with every positive human connection and in turn bonded individuals to the tribe. These days we are more connected to our phones than our tribe. A recent *New York Post* article reported that Americans check their phones eighty times per day on average.

What is tribe in the modern context? We are not wandering the world with our community of thirty to seventy people like we were designed to do. Our modern version of the tribe is our connection to various communities. Maybe you go to church every Sunday and have a few dozen church friends you pray with, or you do CrossFit and have a crew of people there that you suffer with. We are social animals and we will search for groups of people to forge these strong bonds with, even if they are cyber friends. AcroYoga offers good old-fashioned human connection in a way that is timeless and aligned with a healthy sense of self.

PLAY

You can discover more about a person in an hour of play than in a year of conversation.
—PLATO

Play can bring out the most authentic side of us—our inner child. When we play we connect to life in a very full way, and it is the natural progression of human interaction when conditions are safe and fun. Play, laughter, and joy are three key ingredients to improving our quality of life. These feelings do not need to be restricted to when we watch a comedy, do sports, or have sex. It can be a daily practice that AcroYoga activities help to support.

In nature, many animals have a lot of time left over after they have taken care of basic needs, like building shelter or hunting for dinner. If you watch them closely, you will see that they play a lot! In 2018 I had the pleasure of meeting primatologist Isabel Behncke Izquierdo. She shared with me what she witnessed from her years of studying the Bonobo Apes in the Congo. Bonobos play various trust games that to us might seem extreme or a waste of time: It is not

uncommon to see a bigger ape holding a smaller one by the wrist and swinging them from high up in the canopy. The smaller ape does not hold on with their strength, but lets go of fear and trusts the bigger, stronger ape. In this seemingly dangerous act, both apes are laughing and growing their bond. Fun, risk, and trust mix as we learn to find new emotional and physical levels to expand into.

Hunter-gatherer societies also had much more leisure time than we do in our modern lives. Levels of human happiness are much higher when we are doing less and playing more. When you ask a child what they are doing, many times they will give you the same answer—"nothing." In this place of non-doing and being fully present, we engage with life on deeper levels. When we dip our toes into the pool of play there is no room for depression, worry, anger, or the many emotional ailments that plague modern humans. When we play, we win, and we can live life with this aim. What is common to most tribes that still live without modern gadgets and stresses are huge levels of happiness that are unparalleled in any modern society.

Play naturally leads to laughter, and

when we laugh, we communicate many things: "I like you," "I trust you," "I love what we are doing together." Many AcroYogis end up laughing as they do acrobatics, which is challenging because it destabilizes the base and makes all involved train their abs twice as hard! If someone wants to be the best dancer, do they dance the fastest or slowest? Do they dance with a provocative vibe, or is it more about precision? What if the best dancer is the one enjoying it the most? Many fun movements are not based on winning or losing; rather they are done because the act of doing them produces health and happiness. This is the preferred method to train AcroYoga.

Out of all the ways we experience life, smiling and giggling are two things that every human understands. You need no words in common to connect with a group of people laughing and being silly. For all the very complex ways we have developed to relate through culture, language, and rituals, play cuts to the core of human nature and unifies all people, and I can tell you for sure that AcroYoga was born from it: there was very little "work" involved in tapping into the ideas and practices that Jenny and I had in our bodies when we met to play, laugh, jam, experiment, and unlock trust games. Wonderful things can happen when we give ourselves permission to play.

2

THE ROOTS

Acrobatics, Therapeutics, and Yoga

A tree's beauty lies in its branches, but its strength lies in its roots.
—MATSHONA DHLIWAYO

The roots of AcroYoga are three: acrobatics, therapeutics, and yoga. The acrobatic practices are considered "solar," the therapeutic practices "lunar," and the yoga represented by the blend of the solar and lunar practices. They are deep traditions that have evolved independently over time but are surprisingly well suited to one another.

Acrobatics teaches people about risk assessment, goal setting, finding new edges, building trust, and partnership. You need others to grow your acrobatic practice, so by design it grows community, and by doing the practice you grow your relationship skills. Therapeutic practices help us feel our best and address the parts of us that need attention, love, and support. It benefits both the giver and receiver and when done well, both people enter a zen, present, listening state.

From that state many levels of healing and optimization are possible. Knowing how to support the health and healing of others is accessible to all people and will always have value. Finally, yoga is an ancient framework that can give immense depth and direction to everyday life. The accumulation of wisdom from daily practice can help you know more deeply who you are and how you want to live. Yoga helps to balance and align the many layers of your being. Once you understand these three roots, the fusion of AcroYoga will gain more context.

Sometimes, when someone or something new comes into your life, you wonder how you ever survived without them. When I started my journey with therapeutics, I was an acrobat who did some yoga poses, but did not bring breath awareness, compassion, or other layers of yoga to my physical practice. I had a few very substantial gymnastics injuries that gave me a crash course in self-care, self-massage, and healing. But if I knew then what I know now, I would have healed so much faster. The lack of yoga in my formative acrobatics career gave me so much respect and appreciation for the transformational power of yoga when I finally found the practice.

Then when I did, my yoga practice jumped right on the back of my acrobatic control and balance between strength and flexibility. Later I found therapeutics, and that was, and still is, the practice that I think has won me the most friends and that I am most proud of as a tangible contribution to humanity. Learning how to do therapeutic flying and Thai massage has given me a physical, tactile, loving relationship with every person in my blood family and with most of my friends. Being able to express kindness, skill, and love with my touch and acrobatic skills has changed the way I relate to the world and all the people in it.

AcroYoga by design can reach across borders, cultures, and languages. Its roots have many commonalities and some complementary differences. They are all deep practices that can bring more stability to your life and to the people you interact with. From this grounded place, you can decide which branches you want to climb toward, and which fruits interest you the most. Breath, connection, trust, listening, letting go, and many other elements of AcroYoga are present in all three of its root practices. There can be healing present in yoga and in acrobatics, just as there can be acrobatics in yoga and healing. While each of these lineages is unique and profound in its own right, AcroYoga reveals their powerful synergy and compatibility. Read on, practice, and you will see for yourself!

ACROBATICS

Nothing is impossible. The word itself says 'I'm possible.'
—AUDREY HEPBURN

Acrobatics is the flashy, extroverted, solar aspect of AcroYoga. It attracts people like a moth to a flame. In the solar practices of AcroYoga we cultivate fun, communication, clarity, confidence, and presence. Acrobatics challenges and stimulates the body, mind, and emotions of those who do it. People's jaws drop when they see the superhuman feats of strength, flexibility, and balance layered with the risk, trust, and connection between partners. This all started for me in Orangevale, California, at Starz Gymnastics back in 1987. I was twelve when I went to watch my little brother Greg do gymnastics. I liked what I saw, so the next time I went I was not going just to watch—I jumped in! My mom spent the first two hours of my gymnastics career curled over laughing as I fell all over the gym in different ways. For weeks she would come for the entertainment factor of watching me and my brother fumbling around. After a few months the humor gave way to us getting better and more invested. Flipping, swinging, pulling, and pushing my body was my new obsession.

Pre-gymnastics, I was a total Star Wars freak. I had every line memorized and was convinced that I would one day become a Jedi Knight. I would actually close my eyes and try to move objects with my mind. I feel as though I have never stopped training to be one with the Force, and I do believe I am getting closer to becoming a Jedi Master. Way back then, flips and one-armed handstands were all mystical skills that I never knew if I would learn. Many of the gymnastics skills that Luke Skywalker practiced while

studying with Yoda, I eventually learned to do myself. Acrobatics was my Jedi training, and I did learn to move objects with my mind: Acrobats move objects in their minds before their bodies follow suit. I would see the skill, trust myself, my partner, and my coach, and then the Force would take over.

In the practice of acrobatics you focus your mind and body, and through changing both you can reach high levels of precision and union. In this section you will learn about the history and present potential of this magical practice.

The word "acropolis" stems from two roots: *acro,* meaning "on the edge," and *polis,* meaning "city." I have been to Athens many times, and seeing this city perched up on the rocks gives me a very clear illustration of "acro." "Bat" comes from the Greek word βάσκω (*basko:* to go, step, move on foot). Acrobats are people who walk on the edge. By definition you can't do partner acrobatics alone: It is a practice that only exists in community, and the same can be said about AcroYoga. Not only do they walk on the edge, acrobats are also spotted, supported, and coached to do so. They invert, flip, and do things that most people think are impossible. Acrobats practice and expand their awareness and control of their entire body. They do this on all planes of movement: dynamic or static, on their hands or on their feet. They are the ultimate control freaks.

Along with the word "acrobat," the Greeks also gave us the sister movement art of gymnastics. The Ancient Greek word γυμνασία (*gumnasía:* athletic training, exercise) comes from γυμνός (*gumnós:* naked), meaning the Greeks would hang around naked in the gymnasium to philosophize about the world and "swing." They would challenge their bodies as much as their minds.

The main difference between gymnastics and acrobatics is that gymnastics is performed with an apparatus. Men's gymnastics consists of six events: floor exercise, vault, pommel horse, rings, parallel bars, and high bar. Women's gymnastics consists of four events: floor exercise, vault, balance beam, and uneven parallel bars. The competitive discipline of sports acrobatics, where humans become your apparatus, has five events: women's pair, men's pair, mixed pair, women's trio, and men's four.

On the other hand, acrobatics is much less defined. Beyond competitive sports acrobatics there are many circus arts disciplines, and most people who practice

What "acrobatics" means: *to walk on the edge*
How we do it: in partnership, in community, progressively, positively, and safely
Why we do it: to lift each other up

these would likely consider themselves acrobats. Some of these disciplines include trapeze, Chinese pole, straps, tightrope, Spanish web, juggling, Russian swing, teeter board, German wheel, silks, lyra, and the list goes on and on. Over time, we have expanded ancient circus arts and evolved new expressions of acrobatics with breakdancing, figure skating, parkour, pole dancing, surfing, trampoline, and snowboarding, to name just a few. Despite the great variety of disciplines, there is something universal about acrobatic movement: Whether swinging from trees and hunting with spears or playing on jungle gyms and tossing a football, many of our ancient and modern activities can be seen as acrobatic.

Before film was invented there was a boom in circus culture around the world. Circus families trained their children from birth. For job security these circus acrobats would keep their methods secret so they could stay ahead of other acrobats. Even today, despite living in the information age, if you search for resources on acrobatics there is not a big selection. Just as many wisdom traditions are oral, master acrobats passed down their knowledge to students by actually doing acrobatics with them, and students would absorb their skills through direct contact, and trial and error. The wisdom of the practice is contained in the hands and feet of the acrobats who have done the work to earn it experientially.

Traditionally, acrobatics has not been a sport for the masses. It was an elite activity for those born into a circus family, or for children hand-selected by trainers for their exceptional coordination, strength, and bravery. One of the main differences between how AcroYogis and traditional acrobats train is that AcroYoga is inclusive and accessible to all people at all levels of fitness. Now you don't have to run away to join the circus; the circus is most likely playing in your local park with some yoga mats, a slackline, and a bunch of happy people.

Dance, music, and movies all have the potential to thrill and entertain. To move and be moved physically, emotionally, and spiritually are among the essential ingredients of living a full life. Why do

people risk their lives on a daily basis to do acrobatic skills? A very small number of acrobats actually make a living doing it, so it's not for the money. To do acrobatics is an act of becoming fully invested in the present moment. As one goes deeper on the path of becoming an acrobat they experience huge internal shifts. Fear does not disappear, but it decreases as one's ability to know their body's potential, and to assess risk from that place of deep knowing, grows. When people see acrobatics they usually smile, and when you are involved in bringing someone else joy, that is a very magical and gratifying state of being. As you learn to say 'yes' to your own potential you can inspire others to do the same.

There are many ways to train in acrobatics and there are countless forms to try. You can see the acrobatics world as a movement playground with a huge variety of games and principles to discover. These principles can direct your practice no matter what type of acrobatics you are playing with, and they can help you have a better quality of interaction with your partners.

More than anything else, acrobatics is the practice that will change your mind again and again. In the beginning the adult mind says over and over, "I can't do that." As adults we develop so many limiting beliefs that take some work to rewire. Children do not have this limiting mindset; if they see something they like, they assume they can do it and will immediately try it. Many adults have to relearn that open-mindedness. Acrobatics can offer us this potential back. As you build your confidence, the story of "I can't" begins to change to, "Maybe I could try that with a spotter." With even more time, "I could try that" can become, "I bet if we keep at it we'll figure it out." And finally, "Come on, we got this!"

ACROBATIC PRINCIPLES

1. If It's Fun, It's Right.

This is the golden rule for me, and it has to apply to all involved for it to be golden. When you feel safe with your AcroYoga partners, the potential for fun is most present. The safety word in AcroYoga is "down." When we all know that word, we all know there is a clear, easy way out of anything that is not fun anymore. From a grounded place, partners can realign and try again.

I have seen so many acrobats, gymnasts, and other circus performers let these practices be dark and torturous. I decided at a young age that I wanted to do acrobatics because it is fun. As soon as it's not fun for any partner, there is a key pillar out of place. The good news is that when you say 'yes' to acrobatics because you enjoy it, you can sustainably do acrobatics for your whole life.

2. Gravity Is the Teacher.

As much as I like to think I teach people acrobatics, it is not really true. I teach people what I have learned in my own body laboratory as I have traveled the world doing acrobatics. My teacher has always been gravity: She is clear, swift, and constant. When you are aligned well with gravity, her effects are not as strong; when you are misaligned, she will clearly let you know.

3. Bones Are Stronger Than Muscles.

Bones are nature's response to gravity. They do not bend to gravity. In fact, when a load is put on a bone, that stimulation causes more blood to flow in the marrow, increasing bone density and strength. Muscles, on the other hand, are elastic and essential for dynamic power.

Acrobats learn over time to use their muscles to align their bones instead of using only their muscles to do acrobatics. This is called "bone stacking"—when the alignment of the bones supports the weight, and the muscles support the bones to stay in place. When bones take the load of your or your partner's weight, your acrobatic movements will be much more steady, comfortable, and sustainable.

4. Handstand Is the Seed Pose.

In a handstand, you learn to balance your whole body even though you cannot see it. There is a lifelong journey to becoming comfortable and connected to every joint, muscle, and bone in your body and how they work together while you are upside down on your hands.

As flyers progress on their acrobatic path, they practice many variations of handstands on different locations on their base's body. For bases, training in handstands teaches you the same line you will need to find and refine to do standing acrobatics. It helps you understand fear, trust, partnership, and many other aspects vital to the growth of any acrobatic practice. The handstand is the original acrobatic multivitamin.

THERAPEUTICS

The superior doctor prevents sickness; the mediocre doctor attends to impending sickness; the inferior doctor treats actual sickness.
—CHINESE PROVERB

Arguably, health and healing are two of the most important factors in quality of life. Therapeutics will be an important topic for as long as we live. Many of us don't take notice of how we feel until our body demands our attention with pain. We have gone from living and moving in balance with our human design, to changing almost everything we were designed to do: what we eat, our daily movement routines, how much time we spend working, relaxing, and playing. On top of the many imbalances, in the West we have created a reactionary medical system that attempts to cut out or drug our physical symptoms instead of looking at the big picture of our health and our daily lifestyle choices. I have lived a blessed life where I enjoyed the benefits of Western medicine when I was very sick or injured, and Eastern healing traditions for all the other moments of my life. Our anxiety-driven, media-saturated, sedentary modern lifestyles have, on average, taken a big toll on our well-being as a species.

Let's take a look at an average day for someone in the modern workforce in a country like the US. We wake up and go sit on the toilet, then we sit at the table to eat. We eat processed foods full of sugars and chemicals like red #7 that were not a part of our nomadic ancestors' diets. With various forms of caffeine, we throw back our morning calories with haste because we are late to go sit in our cars or on the train, to race to sit at our desk at work. We slam our second cup of coffee and dive into tasks that are oftentimes not meaningful to us or to the ones we love. After our first four hours of sitting we walk to a place to have lunch where we sit again. That walk to lunch was the most natural and healing part of our day so far. After lunch we go back to sitting yet again for another four hours. At many points post-lunch the urge to nap is fierce but unacceptable, so it's back to coffee to help us keep our eye on the target: surviving another workday. Finally, we sit in our cars on the way home and maybe go to the gym where we sit at machines doing very repetitive movements that strengthen our seated patterns with nice-looking muscles.

I know I've painted a very harsh, perhaps even extreme portrait of modern life. But on the other end of this spectrum is the rejection of that lifestyle in favor of one more like the hunter-gatherer societies humans lived in for thousands of years. The simple fact is that, as a species, we are built for daily movement, but most of us no longer engage in a movement lifestyle. The therapeutic branch of AcroYoga addresses this imbalance; it teaches us how to heal ourselves and how to support those around us to experience new levels of balance and well-being.

Let's go back to the beginning. Birth itself is a super intense and wildly beautiful event; it is not uncommon that, in the process, some damage comes to the baby, the mother, or both. We are born into this duality of trauma and healing. To some degree we practice healing and experience new traumas every day until we die. Healing is not something we do only when we are injured or sick. Healing is a daily practice of aligning the many individual pieces of our magnificent bodies in the most optimal way so our lives flow in harmony. It's also something our bodies do in every moment on a cellular level that we cannot easily perceive. There are many ancient and modern perspectives on this topic because

> **What "therapeutic" means:** *to attend to or treat*
> **How we do it:** by listening, loving, and letting go
> **Why we do it:** to slow down, feel better, and give back

we are a complex organism, but there are always principles and patterns from which we can gain understanding. I will present both Western and Eastern ideas about the body, medicine, and healing; between these two traditions, you can build your own therapeutic practices. Central to this approach is the belief that we have many resources in our own bodies and do not need to rely only on doctors and certified healers to fix us. Healing comes in many forms from many people. Massage, dance, cuddling, warm cookies and milk, and a friend that is fully present to hear you are all potential forms of healing for different imbalances. Around the world, AcroYogis practice mindful healing touch and support one another in cultivating wellness through shared presence.

The term "therapeutic" can be traced all the way back to the Greek word *therapeutikos* (from *therapeuein,* meaning "to attend or to treat"). Although the word relates to healing or soothing, "therapeutic" isn't reserved only for drugs or medical treatments. You've probably heard particular activities referred to as therapeutic, which just means doing those activities makes you feel rejuvenated. These softer practices range from but are not limited to Thai massage, AcroYoga flying, and partner yoga. They are designed to complement the fire of the solar acrobatic practices. As AcroYogis, movement, connection, and play are our first lines of defense in the battle against pain, suffering, and disconnection. The word "healing" comes from the Old English word *harlan,* meaning "to make whole." Health and wellness have become huge topics of modern political debate as more of the global population suffers from disease and depression each year. Some companies are beginning to invest significant resources in their employees' wellness as it is becoming clear that the health or sickness of their staff has a direct impact on the health of the company.

The body itself is always doing everything it can to support your life. We do many random, crazy things to our bodies each day, and like a loyal dog the body comes back wagging its tail, ready for whatever we throw its way. It is inevitable that there will be moments of ease, flow, and connection among all of the different parts of you, and it's also

guaranteed that disconnection, disease, and pain will be part of your human experience too. Listening to your own body, and learning to listen to others as a healing practitioner, are the doorways to many healing states. Where attention goes, energy flows. If we are feeling compassion, and if our partner feels compassion in our touch, we are already co-creating a healing space for both people. Healing is not done or performed "on" a person—it's a collaborative process. There are practices to offer stretching, compression, traction, and connection, and there are practices to bring heat and blood to support the body's inherent vitality.

On an emotional and energetic level, there are practices to communicate compassion through touch. I want to offer a brief view into healing from different perspectives and then share how they contribute to AcroYoga. Healing ourselves is as natural as hurting ourselves. When we stub our toe we all know what to do: We yell something unsavory in our mother tongue, jump around a bit to release all the extra energy that surged through our nervous system, and on the other side we hold our toe with a soft, loving touch. There are variations on this theme for sure, but the basic premise holds:

We do not need to go to medical school or become a massage therapist to heal ourselves or others. It has been part of our human blueprint forever. Similarly, loving-kindness is a quality we are all capable of, and it has huge benefits both for the person who feels it for someone else, and for the person for whom this feeling is generated. It is one of the quintessential win-win dynamics that humans can co-create.

In early times, mysticism, shamanism, and local herbs were our main sources of healing. Over time these ways were tested by generations of people, and the ancient medical traditions of the world took form. Ayurveda is a medicine system from India that translates to "the science of life," or "the complete knowledge for long life." Ayurveda sees people as having a disposition to certain balances and imbalances in their constitution, or *dosha*. The three *doshas* are *Vata, Pitta,* and *Kapha*. These constitutions are based on the elements of earth, water, fire, air, and ether. On a very simplistic level, depending on your *dosha*, certain foods and practices will either balance you or bring you more out of balance. Yoga and Ayurveda are sister sciences and they share a great deal of foundational concepts. As one learns to apply the sciences of both yoga and Ayurveda together, they are practicing yoga therapy. The way I chose the elements of yoga to incorporate into AcroYoga was based on this idea of complementary practices. In AcroYoga the dynamic nature of acrobatics complements the gentle nature of therapeutics.

THE ENERGY BODY

Beneath all our muscles and bones there is a nervous system. Beneath all our matter there is a soul. These are all words to speak about your energy body. *Prana* is the Sanskrit word for "life force" and *Qi* is the Chinese word for "energy"—what flows through the energetic superhighway of your body. Masters of yoga, qigong, marshal arts, and acrobatics all know how to move energy. Science tells us we cannot create or destroy energy, rather it changes from one state to another. The mystics, sages, and meditators from India say there are 72,000 *nadis,* or energy channels, in the body. From that total count, there are larger pathways called *vayus* or "wind channels." These are energetic rivers where life force flows.

Sometimes in life our *prana* gets blocked; this could mean blood is not flowing to certain tissues, there are knots in your muscles, your nervous system is overloaded, or you have limiting beliefs. There are both obvious and subtle ways to remove blockages. Both are needed and both have immense value. Imagine your body as a piece of bamboo. When we experience *pranic* blockages, it's like getting dirt stuck in the middle of the bamboo—no wind can flow through it. You can bang the bamboo from the outside with a big stick, or you can take a little stick and poke at the dirt from the inside. In this analogy, the big stick represents strong physical movements such as running, jumping, yoga asana (physical postures), and massage. The little stick represents the subtle-body practices like meditation, breathwork, taking a bath, singing, sleeping, and praying. Over time, mindful practice can empower you to direct your flow of energy and vitality into different parts of your body, thereby steering your health and healing.

Traditional Chinese Medicine (TCM) is a very well tested, ancient system that has supported people for thousands of years. There are many parallels between the Indian and Chinese healing arts traditions. They both recognize energetic systems in the body. In TCM the channels are called *meridians*. Both traditions also hold balance as foundational. In yoga, the practice of physical balance is called *Hatha*, *ha* meaning "sun" and *tha* meaning "moon." In TCM balance is represented by the yin-yang symbol, a black-and-white circle with two dots. Just as in Ayurveda, there are five elements that relate our human condition to nature, but in TCM those elements are earth, fire, water, wood, and metal. As amazing as modern medicine is, there is a simple elegance to the ancient systems, and the power of blending both ancient and modern medicine is what we are capable of in today's healing landscape.

Since the scientific revolution in the sixteenth century, humanity has been steadily shifting more focus and trust in healing to doctors and scientists. With the support of science, innovations in hygiene and surgical technique have changed medicine forever. One of the realities of this system is that it is very analytical, meaning that mystical or spiritual experiences "unproven" by science have, to a large degree, been dumped like a bad prom date. Whatever your current beliefs are, more Eastern or Western, there is value in seeing your health from different perspectives. With this new well-rounded view you can apply the right system at the right time to support your well-being.

When most people think of medicine, they think of pills and surgeries. *Allopathic medicine* refers to modern science-based treatments such as the use of medications and surgical procedures to treat or suppress symptoms of disease. If my appendix ruptures, I do not want someone to rub essential oils on my belly and chant mantras. I want anesthesia, a sharp scalpel, and a well-trained surgeon. Each practice has its brilliance. Fixing someone when they are broken is a valid practice, but I also like to think of health and medicine as a question of lifelong balance. In Chinese medicine, elements are either in excess or deficient, full or empty. With different treatments you can tonify, or build up, *qi* (energy) in areas that are deficient, or reduce *qi* in areas with an excess.

While all healing practitioners have different tools and modalities, to a large degree the practice of offering therapeutics connects the different systems of the body that are not in harmony and finds ways to balance them. Healers connect through touch and are supreme listeners. To heal you must get in touch with yourself, your intentions, and nature. As you fine-tune your ability to listen, you will meet your needs and the needs of others more deeply.

THERAPEUTIC PRINCIPLES

1. If It Feels Good, It's Right.

Win-win situations are the best way to build trust and make friends. If as a giver you feel good, you can give so much more. If as a receiver you feel good, you are honoring your needs.

In every moment we can and should align with this principle, and any time things do not feel good or right, the next step is communicating so a new alignment can be found.

2. Gravity Is the Therapist.

A lifetime of learning to move against and with gravity can build up many structural imbalances and holding patterns in the body. When we hang passively in therapeutic flying, we can let gravity realign us with our optimal spinal blueprint.

To be sustainable in how we offer therapeutic treatments of any kind, we must find the techniques that allow gravity to do the work rather than overworking our muscles. As we learn to soften our points of contact, the receiver's body has a greater potential to receive transformational benefits.

3. Body Comfortable.

This is the one principle I have given the most attention to in my career as a healer and a teacher of healing arts. It seems simple because it is. Like most simple things, within this principle is infinite complexity.

Because tissues can sense tissues, if you lightly touch skin to skin, they recognize each other. If you apply more pressure, the muscles feel and recognize each other. If you push bone on bone, they recognize each other too, and it is not a fun feeling.

If as you are giving treatments you are listening to your body, you will feel which tissues are playing nice together. If you are not comfortable in your contact points, likely neither is your receiver.

From the micro of therapeutics to the macro of your life, this principle can guide your state of being most of the time. You simply need to give your attention to what you feel, and have the courage to make changes, especially in how you relate to others.

4. Movement Is Life, Stagnation Is Death.

If doctors had only one prescription for the whole of humanity— one habit to dedicate to for life—I believe this miracle drug would be movement. Our bodies are dynamic systems that need to be used to be at their optimal potential.

Personally, I know many people between the ages of sixty and eighty-five years old that are very healthy and capable. What they all have in common is that they have never stopped their movement practices. "Use it or lose it" is not a theory, it's a basic law of life, and these people prove it.

Like in nature, when water moves it is vital, pure, and full of life. When water stagnates, it easily gets polluted and becomes a breeding ground for disease and death.

YOGA

What did the yogi say to the hot dog vendor?

"Make me one with everything!"

The hot dog vendor did just that and received a fresh twenty-dollar bill from the yogi.

The yogi asked impatiently, "What about my change?"

The hot dog vendor replied with a big smile, "Change comes from within."

I love this joke because it's one of the few I remember and it lightens up the sometimes heavy topic of spirituality and yoga. In 2007 I did my first AcroYoga world tour, taking this very young, unknown practice to many new places. One of those places was India. Before I arrived, *Time Out Mumbai* magazine heard we were coming and decided to do an article about AcroYoga. In the phone interview they asked some interesting questions: "It seems from the photos on your website that people enjoy doing AcroYoga and even laugh when your yoga is performed. What do you think the Indian yogis will think of that?" I responded, "Uh, I think they will like it." To me it seemed normal that fun and yoga would go hand in hand, because that is how I designed AcroYoga. But in India at that time, yoga was still something your grandfather did and it was nothing to smile about. Many people in the West share this austere attitude. While self-discipline and mastery are worthy attributes, they can easily tip over into a sense of arrogance and superiority. I have heard many people say that AcroYoga is not "real" yoga, precisely because it is fun, playful, and involves interaction with others. But "yoga" means union, or connection. What could be more "yogic" than connecting with others to create something greater than ourselves?

The partnership element of AcroYoga definitely makes it more fun, but it also challenges you to take the work you have done on your own yoga mat and the wisdom you have gained in self-reflection and put them into practice in your relationships, your community, and the way you show up in the world. Because of the emphasis it places on communication and relationships, some have described AcroYoga as "the yoga of trust."

FEAR, JOY, AND TRUST

Let's look at fear. We all have it, some more than others. Fear is not good or bad, it is simply a part of our human experience. What can be beneficial about fear is when it slows us down and demands high degrees of mindfulness. What can be detrimental about fear is when it paralyzes us and keeps us living life in a very small range of possibilities. I see fear as potential joy, and I excel at helping convert people's fear into joy. The catalyst for this transformation is trust. Trust is the invisible hand that nudges someone along this spectrum of potential. These elements are more common to AcroYoga than traditional yoga due to the partner work and edges you inevitably end up meeting and exploring in the practice.

Yoga can be many things to many people, and as its popularity continues to grow worldwide it will surely evolve into many more variations in the years to come. At its core, it is a sacred and ancient practice with traceable origins and time-honored principles that are as fundamental to AcroYoga as they are to any other modern yoga practice. One of the things I admire most about yoga

What "yoga" means: *union or connection*
How we do it: consistently, patiently, with daily and lifelong practices
Why we do it: to know, love, and evolve thyself

is how adaptable it is as a system: It has proven that, over hundreds of years and across different cultures and societies, it can be adapted to fit into very different lives and lifestyles, and contributes to a sense of balance, well-being, and harmony in all of them. The sufferings and traumas we encounter in life can make us rigid and edgy. Yoga is a practice to smooth out our edges and bring us back to the simple miracles of breath, movement, and gratitude.

Yoga is a Sanskrit word meaning "to join, yoke, or unify." It is another word for connection, and can be elaborated as the union of body, mind, and spirit; the union of masculine and feminine; the union of the self to the universal divine. Yoga is famous for its ability to transform people on many levels. In the West, most people who practice yoga start out with a posture practice focused on the body. But over time yoga can end up altering everything from one's daily routines, digestion, and quality of sleep, to one's entire outlook and attitude toward life. This is the power of connection: from a place of yoga or "union," we can enhance our skills in true discernment and understanding, optimal alignment, self-knowledge, and peace. This simple four-letter word is quite expansive, and there are countless variations of yoga today being practiced all over the world.

FROM EAST TO WEST: THE MIGRATION OF YOGA

How did this ancient practice make it from India around the world? It was not by accident. There were pioneers who set out to codify and expand modern yoga, and "yoga missionaries" who brought these teachings out of India and across the globe. Among the most important pioneers was Tirumalai Krishnamacharya, a yogi, Ayurvedic healer, and scholar who was born in 1888 in what is now Karnataka, Southern India. Often referred to as "the father of modern yoga," Krishnamacharya is widely regarded as one of the most influential yoga teachers

of the twentieth century. He blended different movement practices as a disciple of the ancient yogic and Ayurvedic traditions. He also drew on European athletics culture, particularly gymnastics, as he developed his own unique system. At his *shala* in Mysore, he trained an army of yogis who would go on to spread his teachings around the world.

Krishnamacharya's students included many of yoga's most renowned and influential teachers: Indra Devi, T. K. V. Desikachar (his son), and K. Pattabhi Jois, the founder of Ashtanga yoga. B. K. S. Iyengar, the founder of Iyengar yoga, also credits Krishnamacharya with introducing him to yoga as a boy in the 1930s. All of these renowned teachers— the heavyweights of "global yoga" in the twentieth century—would have been familiar with something similar to AcroYoga. This is because we know, from photographs and films taken in the 1930s, that Krishnamacharya "flew" his students in aerial postures instantly recognizable to any modern AcroYogi.

Yoga has truly lived up to its name by connecting each corner of the modern world. In America, yoga is predominantly a form of fitness, while in India it is often practiced by singing sacred mantras toward various Gods. Both are examples of yoga, and both are about connection. For over five thousand years the practices of yoga have been cultivated and passed from guru to disciple throughout India. The beginning of the twentieth century is when many gurus decided to send their best students out into the world to share their discoveries. These discoveries are philosophies and daily practices that can improve one's health, wellness, and balance. Sounds good, right? It is, and that is why it's so popular. Yoga changes people's lives.

WHERE ACRO MEETS YOGA

On a physical level, solo yogis use their own muscles to push their bodies into poses. As anyone who has ever had a great assist from a yoga teacher can tell you, there are many things you can do with a partner that you simply cannot do by yourself. By the simple fact that we are doing partner work and usually balancing each other's bodies, AcroYogis are pulled into the present moment and obliged to give their whole attention to the task at hand. When doing partner yoga one person can be like a yoga prop, allowing the other to relax over their support. The weight of another person can also help open the body by adding more force than one person has alone. Specifically when basing, the weight of an entire human rests on your legs; this warms and strengthens the muscles, and can help unlock new ranges of flexibility in a very short time.

You might be very good at yoga on your mat, in a yoga studio, with incense burning and nice music, but how are you in traffic, or at Thanksgiving dinner with your whole family? As you learn to apply yoga to your relationships, you can become more skilled at finding and maintaining harmony with yourself and others. AcroYogis who choose to grow their yoga practice have some huge advantages. Solo yoga practices help us check in with ourselves and continue the process of individual evolution. Then in partnership, we get to practice being a bigger, better version of ourselves with others who are also invested in our growth and well-being.

Many people have a very small circle of true support: if we're lucky, we have family, a spouse, or a best friend. When you find partners in AcroYoga, you automatically gain cheerleaders who want to see you do well and will ideally also call you out on your shit. You being the best version of yourself makes your partnership stronger, so getting honest feedback about how you are showing up is an invaluable gift. If you don't like the feedback, maybe you end the partnership and find a new, nicer AcroYogi. But after a few weeks when the same triggers come up, you may get the same feedback that your last partner gave you. In reality, the whole community can act as a support system and shine praise on you when you show up in an authentic way. They can also bring you back to earth if your interactions are consistently leading to negative places for yourself and the community members around you.

In the modern world, where doing more and doing it faster is the common trend, yoga helps us slow things down and focus on the present moment. It is a practice that can increase our awareness of who we are and what we can do on a daily basis to live more fulfilled lives. Is yoga a spiritual practice, a religion, or a workout? "Yes" is my answer, and like all things it depends on the intention of the practitioner. The type of yoga

most famous around the world is called *hatha yoga*. It is the "gateway drug" to many other addictive yoga practices. These other practices can range from cleansing the body, practicing non-violence, being truthful, meditation, prayer, breathwork, chanting the names of Hindu gods, focusing the mind, non-attachment, studying ancient texts, dietary changes, opening the energy centers of the body, and others.

So maybe you have a yoga mat and know a few poses. What else are you practicing that is bringing more to the table than flexibility and deeper breathing? Yogis work to align their thoughts, words, and actions. In the pursuit of a balanced, happy life, ancient yogis distilled and described a clear moral code to help others reach more peace and maybe even moments of enlightenment. One of the most influential books on yoga is called the *Yoga Sūtras of Patañjali*. This sacred text was written around 400 CE. It is not known where Sri Patañjali lived, or even if he was a single person or rather several persons using the same title. Whoever he/they were, Patañjali synthesized and organized the knowledge of yoga from other texts and masters to create a one-stop yoga bible. This book gave practitioners a single place to deepen their understanding of themselves and study practices to help them control their mind. Yoga is a vast science and most people know about *hatha yoga*, the physical yoga practice; much of this book is focused on *raja yoga*, the yoga of the mind. The following principles are my offering to you as you step deeper into this mystical, magical, and practical world of body, mind, and spirit connection.

PRINCIPLES OF YOGA

1. Cultivate Daily Practices.

Contemporary mystic and yogi Jaggi Vasudev, known publicly as Sadhguru, says, "Everything can be *sādhanā*. The way you eat, the way you sit, the way you stand, the way you breathe, the way you conduct your body, mind, and your energies and emotions— this is *sādhanā*."

Sādhanā is the Sanskrit word for "practice." What is unique to the practice of yoga is that everything can become a part of your practice. Setting intentions, meditation, prayer, and even things like going for a walk, steeping tea, or growing a garden can all be considered yogic practices when done mindfully.

Humans in ancient cultures were steeped in rituals through their daily routines. Modern culture is much more transactional and devoid of these simple but potent practices, and we must learn to bring them back in order to experience the true potential of yoga. There is no magic potion to becoming a more amazing version of yourself—the practice itself is the magic potion.

2. Poses Can Be Steady and Comfortable.

Sthira sukhamasanam.
—YOGA SUTRAS OF PATANJALI, 2.45

Sthira is a Sanskrit word that may be translated as "steadiness" or "strength." This word comes from the root word *stha*, which means "to stand" or "to be firm." *Asthi*, meaning "bone," is another root word that offers clues to this Sanskrit riddle for steadiness. These words collectively imply resolution, courage, and firmness.

To feel this in action, do a plank pose with straight arms for five breaths and feel the physical and emotional quality of finding the bone layer. Next, do a plank with your arms bent. This aggravating, fiery sensation is the muscular layer. If we stay in the muscles too long we shake, and then we get emotionally and physically unsettled.

Sukham means "easy." When we find alignment through our bones we can plug into the earth with ease. This is another way you can evaluate your progress in different poses.

As the body gets stronger, more flexible, and more skilled, the poses that used to be hard become easier and easier. This focus on the quality of the practice is central to the gift of yoga. Yoga is about learning how to find and observe the right level of depth in your postures where you can still breathe, smile, and enjoy.

3. Be Attached to Non-attachment.

This principle is cheeky in hopes that you remember it. Yoga is a practice of transformation and for it to be consistent, we must be brave enough to let go.

But wait a minute! You just said, "Do your daily rituals." Now let go of that? Paradoxes are where most of the interesting parts of life live. Say 'yes' to rituals, and to practice, but also say 'yes' to letting go of them and finding new ones as the seasons inevitably change.

THREE IS THE MAGIC NUMBER

Once upon a time there was a prince named Ram. Ram was in love with Sita, the most beautiful princess in all the land. To win Sita's hand in marriage there was a competition to string Lord Shiva's bow. Ravana, a demon king from another land, desperately wanted to have Sita as his wife. Many potential suitors came to compete, but Ram was the only one who had the power to string the bow and he won Sita's hand in marriage. Ravana was not happy with this outcome and vowed that Sita would one day be his. Not long after, Sita and Ram were in the forest when Ravana showed up and used his sorcery to kidnap Sita. Ram was devastated.

Elsewhere in the forest lived a monkey god named Hanuman who was soon to be Ram's best friend. Hanuman was a very sweet, playful creature who had been granted many superhuman powers he could only access from a place of service. He saw the suffering in Ram and offered to lend him support. This offer would lead him on an epic adventure that included jumping from mainland India all the way to Sri Lanka. This is why the splits are called *hanumanasana* in yoga. He jumped into this pose, flew across the sea, and eventually saved the day, rescuing Sita from her captor.

There are many details I am leaving out of this elaborate Hindu tale, of course, but what is key to this story and how it relates to AcroYoga is the concept of three people supporting one another to become the best versions of themselves. There is the base, Ram, who is strong, stable, and able to lift and support the flyer. There is the flyer, Sita, who faces many fears but is trusting because she feels the support of her base. And then there is the spotter, Hanuman, who is there to offer his service when needed. The spotter's role is to strengthen the relationship between the base and flyer. By no means do bases need to be alpha males, flyers beautiful princesses, or spotters monkey gods. AcroYoga by design is for all people, and switching roles provides the best platform for understanding, learning, and compassion. Three is the magic number for so many reasons, and I will point out many of them in this chapter. Base, flyer, and spotter is the smallest community in AcroYoga. This triad is what is needed to progress safely and to give you the tools to further build community. Let's look at how our brains work in a dualistic world first, and then examine how we can shift our point of view from dualism to the magic of three.

To do as well as we have as a species, we needed to survive scores of challenges over countless generations. In this time our brains evolved a highly developed frontal lobe. This is the part of our brain that classifies things, helps us problem solve, and allows us to think into the future. One of my yoga scholar friends calls this type of reasoning the "yum-yuck" duality. We either like something

or we don't. We can eat it or it can eat us. This ability to understand the risks and opportunities in front of us has been a key part of us reaching our evolutionary potential. As we have come out of the caves and into modern life, we now have the potential to evolve our worldview. Instead of a dualistic world of good and bad, we can practice seeing a three-dimensional world where there are two poles to any given topic and a third aspect in between. This third aspect is the wisdom that you gather as you move from one pole to the other.

When considering duality, it is important to note that "positive" and "negative" are not to be confused with good and bad. One cannot exist without the other. The north pole and south pole are both cool and interesting; one is not better than the other. Because of their polarity, there exists a magnetic field that shields our entire planet from the harsh radiation of space. Countless species utilize this magnetic field to navigate their long migrations. The power of magnetism is supported by polarity, and we can discover it when we explore between the poles.

MAGIC OF THREE

POSITIVE	NEGATIVE	NEUTRAL
Yang	Yin	Tao
Sun	Moon	Yoga
Strength	Flexibility	Balance
Red	Blue	Purple

In the previous pages I explored acrobatics, therapeutics, and yoga. In the pages that follow I will continue with other triads that will help you get the most out of learning and practicing AcroYoga. In Chapter 5 you will find the AcroYoga Table of Elements, where I have laid out the many physical forms of the practice. This table also contains what I call the Noble Elements—the universal qualities that students develop as they practice AcroYoga—regardless of age, gender, or background. As you will see, these qualities are also organized in triads.

I dedicated a decade of my life to traveling the world spreading AcroYoga and in that time I learned how it affects different people from different cultures. I have made some amazing and unexpected discoveries about the nature of human beings. I remember so clearly wondering before my first world tour, *What will a Chinese 'om'*

sound like, and *What will an Indian 'om' sound like?* As it turns out, om is om and people are people! All the people I have worked with have had surprisingly similar responses to doing AcroYoga. People love it! It makes them smile and laugh no matter what country they are from. Of course there are some cultural differences: In Japan as soon as class is over, students immediately go to scrub their mats clean. In some parts of the Middle East and India, mixed-gender AcroYoga classes are less permissible due to religious and cultural views.

But once people get hooked, they find the potential to infuse their existing way of life with AcroYoga's unique perspective on the world. When you are doing AcroYoga well, the Noble Elements are the qualities and states of being that you enjoy. The full body-mind-spirit integration possible with AcroYoga can only be actualized by actually doing it; in truth, I believe this is the reason why many people fall in love with the practice.

Here I will share the Noble Elements, you will see them again in different chapters. In the first column are the Noble Elements of acrobatics in red, from the hook of fun to the ability to be present. The blue boxes in the second column are those of therapeutics,

NOBLE ELEMENTS OF ACROYOGA

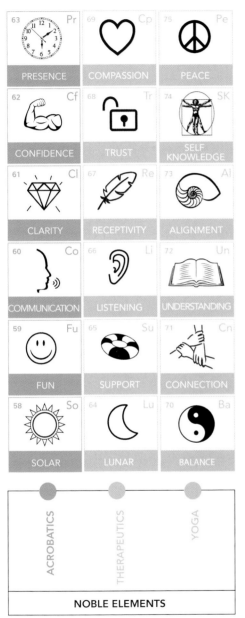

from our desire to exchange support to the gift of compassion. Lastly, those elements in the purple boxes of the third column are cultivated in yoga, from the seed of connection to the flower of peace. They are sequentially ordered from obvious and easy to experience at the bottom, to subtle and more difficult to sustain at the top.

Fun, support, and connection are the foundation from which the practice grows. You cannot do AcroYoga without support and connection, and if it's not fun, you are definitely not doing it right! Being present, compassionate, and at peace might be easy to experience for a moment, but they are also easy to lose awareness of. The triads in the Noble Elements are found as you progress from left to right: by mixing a solar element with a lunar element, you discover the yogic element. For example, as you mix communication with listening, you find understanding. When you have clarity of what you want and receptivity in how to get there, you can find alignment.

The next step in this book is getting you ready for your first flight. This requires understanding of the three roles in AcroYoga. Once equipped with that knowledge, I will share with you how to get in the air.

THE THREE ROLES OF ACROYOGA: BASE, FLYER, AND SPOTTER

Three is the magic number in AcroYoga because the trio of base, flyer, and spotter is what you need to safely get your practice off the ground. This is the smallest AcroYoga community. This magical constellation inherently nurtures progress, stability, and safety, and what you learn in this group of three can be scaled to bigger groups.

You might have had your first flight from your parents years ago with "airplane." This section is designed to get you back flying the friendly skies with a friend you know or with friends you haven't met yet. We play acro because it's fun. Safety helps us sustain the fun, and for AcroYoga to be safe we must have agreements about the physical techniques and how we communicate. It's time to put our phones down and lift each other up!

The Base

Let's start with our foundation—the base. The base is the one that creates the platform for the AcroYoga to happen. Their stability supports the flyer in being lifted and freed from the clutches of gravity. A base is supported or limited by their own awareness of their body and how they communicate and listen. A great base is a very clear communicator and an even better listener. Basing entails listening with your feet, hands, bones, and eyes. Strength is a component for sure, but using strength to find alignment in the bones is even more powerful.

The Flyer

Next is the flyer. The flyer has the pleasure of being lifted and supported. Smiles, giggles, and happy dances often come from the flyer. They take more risks and also enjoy more attention. The skill of the flyer is, to a large degree, dependent on how well they can lean into the base's support, know when to say "down," and when to ask for a spotter.

The Spotter

Completing the triad is the spotter. The spotter is the magician in the trio who wields the most subtle and nuanced skills. Their support helps people experience pivotal breakthroughs, yet they will hardly ever get an Instagram post. The spotter's first responsibility is their own safety, then the flyer's safety. Once safe, the spotter's outside eye can support the base's alignment. Spotters are invited guests to the base-flyer party. They should do the minimum, and when they are doing a great job you will know it because they will catch the flyer at crucial moments when you hardly noticed they were there. With this triad you can safely attempt and have success in many realms of the practice.

Practice All Roles

What you learn as you change roles from base to flyer and then to spotter is to have compassion for other people. It is natural and common to be more interested or invested in a certain role; having dedicated partners in dedicated roles is an amazing step to developing a more advanced practice. But to really get the most out of AcroYoga, it is good on a regular basis to step out of your customary role and learn firsthand what your partner usually experiences. Feel the fear of flying, know the challenge of being a stable base, and learn the power of supporting your friends as you get better at spotting. These steps away from your usual tendencies can increase your compassion and clarity in the type of partner you want to be.

As we gain the courage to step out of our comfort zones we can learn so much more about what others go through. This is how the global AcroYoga community has been formed since 2003, and by this time millions of people have been brave enough to meet strangers and treat them like family. They all exchange trust, support, and presence as if they were invisible currencies. AcroYoga is designed for all types of people, and you can and will find others who will be honored and excited to join you in your next steps into this beautiful world of co-created play. Now that you know the roles, it's time to get ready for your first flight!

4

YOUR FIRST FLIGHT

There are many things we learn from our parents that they learned from theirs, and as a society we blindly accept many philosophies. One of the lessons I learned as a kid was, "Don't talk to strangers." I know there are fears about unknowns, and there are some people in the world who will harm you and the ones you love. All of that being present and true, treating every person in the world who you don't know with a cold indifference has a huge cost.

Given that I have the tools to fly people and gain their trust, I have flown literally thousands of strangers and become friends with them. I have also seen the people I've trained do the same. It is so much fun helping people trust and play with strangers. This is one of the most meaningful things about AcroYoga, so I will spend the next several pages setting you and your friends up for a fun and life-changing first flight. With enough experience, you will then be able to share this with anyone.

These step-by-step instructions will help you build your AcroYoga practice as a base, flyer, and spotter. If you have always wondered what you are truly capable of, or want to impress your friends at the next party, this section will fill your bag of tricks with many new AcroYoga moves.

PRE-FLIGHT CHECKLIST

Before you take off in a plane, emergency procedures are always announced. In AcroYoga, knowing the proper safety measures improves the overall comfort and success of your flight. While exact etiquette varies, the following points serve as a good baseline:

- » If it's fun for all involved, it's right.
- » Help your base up and down from the floor.
- » Listen to your body and ask for what you need.
- » Down means down. It's the AcroYoga "safety word."
- » The base, flyer, or spotter can call "down" at any time—and when you hear it, immediately help the flyer return to the ground.

Get Ready to Fly!

In the following pages I will lead you toward doing one of the most important, essential and well-known flying poses—Front Plank (FP). Each exercise in this four-step progression will teach you skills that will build your ability to do harder and more exciting poses.

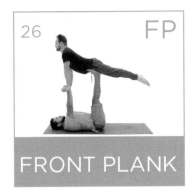

FRONT PLANK

The process of calibrating with your partners is as valuable as the actual skill toward which you are building, so take the time to try these exercises with your partner before jumping right to flying.

Plan Your Intinerary: Find Your Stack, Know Your Actions

» **Find Your Stack:**
  To find ease in AcroYoga you must learn to align the geometry of your bones with gravity. This is called 'bone stacking' and it will almost always include finding straight and vertical lines through the legs of the base and the arms of both the base and flyer. We are looking for skyscraper vertical versus Leaning Tower of Pisa diagonal.

» **Know Your Primary Actions:**
  Set yourself up for success by learning to clarify the most important actions of a skill you are attempting. By identifying what movements you will need to make in order to accomplish the skill, you will have taken the first step toward embodying the pose.

  For the base doing a Front Plank (FP), the primary action is bending and extending the arms and legs. The flyer's primary actions are squeezing muscles to unify the body and pouring their weight into the points of contact the base is offering.

1. Find Your Lines: Plank on Plank

Let's begin with finding your stack. Step One in our progression will give you confidence, clarify your technique, and probably make one or both of you smile! You will stack one Plank (Pl) on top of the other and in the process discover the importance of bone stacking, or vertically aligning your bones to find stability.

» The **base places their hands** under their shoulders with straight arms; feet are the flyer's shoulder width apart.

» Flyer **checks that the base's arms are vertical** and feet shoulder width of the flyer.

» Flyer **holds the base's ankles**, thumbs in, fingers out and lifts **one foot at a time** to the base's upper back, the tops of their feet facing down.

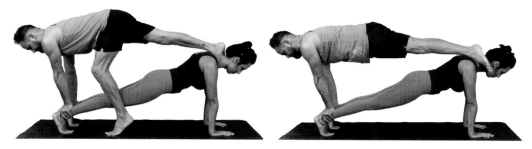

Flyer Places One Foot at a Time   Plank on Plank

» Once up, both base and flyer hold their shape and feel the **stability through the arms** and rest of their bodies.

2. **Test Flight: L-Base Alignment Drill**

L-basing is the term for when a base performs AcroYoga lying down with their legs vertical. Their body creates an L shape, hence the name L-base. Before you fly it's a good idea to test your base's ability to straighten their legs in their L shape while supporting weight. This drill helps the base find bone stacking in their legs.

» **Base presents their legs vertically** with feet hip width apart.

» Flyer places their **forearms on the base's feet** and pushes down.

» Next the **flyer lifts their feet**, offering their full bodyweight to test the base's ability to keep their legs vertical and straight.

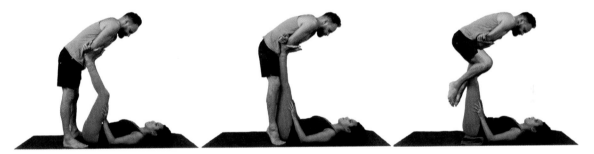

Help Base Find Alignment   Legs Straight, Flyer Pushes Down   Flyer Offers All Their Weight

» If the **base cannot keep their legs straight** or vertical, you can allow for a slight bend in the base's knees by **folding up a yoga mat** or towel to place under the base's hips. This will make basing easier while they build up their flexibility over time. If the base is more comfortable with their leg alignment, the flyer will have a better time in the air.

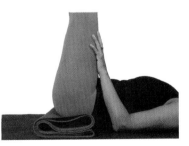

Optional Mat Support for Base

Now Boarding! Set Your Foundation

Now that you've found stability in your Plank poses, and tested your base's leg alignment, it's time to get set up to fly. Before we take flight in AcroYoga, we must learn how our bodies fit together with hand grips and foot placements. Knowing these contact points is essential, so let's start with our foundation.

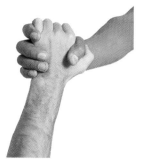

Reverse Hand to Hand Grip
from Flyer Point of View

» **Reverse Hand to Hand Grip:**
The flyer presents their hands with their fingers facing forward. Think "FFF": Flyer's Fingers Forward.

The base presents their hands with fingers turned out.

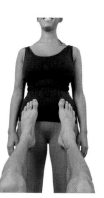

Front Plank (FP) Foot
Placement

» **Front Plank (FP) Foot Placement:**
Base's feet are approximately hip width and parallel, their heels at the tops of the flyer's thighs and their toes pointed toward the belly of the flyer.

The flyer's hip bones should be in the middle of the base's feet. If the feet are in the right place, it should be easy for the base to support the flyer and comfortable for the flyer.

3. **Prepare for Take Off: Front Plank (FP) Prep**

   This exercise will train the two keys you'll need for the pose: the foundation and the action.

   The foundation is the base's feet parallel, heels at the tops of the flyer's thighs, toes pointed toward the flyer's belly. The flyer's hip bones should be at the middle of each foot.

   The base's action is bending and straightening the legs, and the flyer's action is squeezing their body and holding the plank shape.

» The **flyer stands close to the base** in a Plank (Pl) shape with their hands facing the base.

» Without the flyer changing shape, the **base bends their legs** until they can touch the flyer's hands.

» The **base then presses back** to extended.

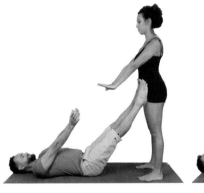 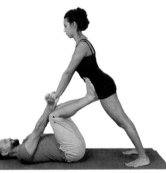 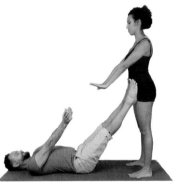

Base's Feet at Flyer's Hips   Base Bends Legs   Base Extends Legs

» Repeat, **making any needed adjustments** in the base's foot placement or distance between the flyer and base.

4. Buckle Up! It's Time to Fly: Front Plank (FP) aka "Airplane"

Having tried all the preparatory poses, this will be an easy and logical next step. Make sure the base has the padding they need if they struggle to keep legs straight and vertical.

» **Flyer sets up in their Front Plank** (FP) position with base's feet parallel at their hips, flyer's fingers facing forward.

» Both partners look at each other, take a deep breath, and exhale as **base bends their legs until they connect hands** with the flyer.

» Once their hands connect, the base bends their arms, and the flyer holds their arms and **whole body straight and tight**.

» When the flyer's weight is over the base's center, the base extends their arms and legs until they **find vertical lines** through both.

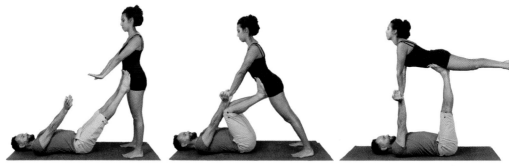

Base's Feet at Flyer's Hips   Base Bends Legs   Front Plank (FP)

» Your **spotter is at the side** with one hand under the flyer's belly and the other arm under their legs. Flyer keeps looking forward and squeezing their muscles. Both base and flyer keep their arms straight and vertical.

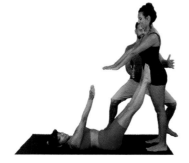
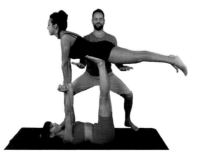

With Spotter   Spotter Moves with Flyer

PART II
SMART TRAINING

There are so many ways to train in movement arts. Because AcroYoga is a partner practice, it is even more complex than solo practices. There is no machine in a gym that can offer you the stabilizing muscles and agility needed to balance a human. New skills can be hard at first, but what you always have in AcroYoga is the support of your partners.

When done intelligently AcroYoga can be a lifelong practice. AcroYoga moms and dads fly and play with their children from day one, and I have seen many grandparents enjoy the gift of flight too. The learning and growing never end, and each person will need you to show up in different and unique ways to get the most out of your training with them.

I have designed the next section to show you the key elements of training and building your AcroYoga skills so you can enjoy the fullness of this practice. Seeing the Table of Elements, learning the art of training, and incorporating new ways to increase your strength and flexibility will create the best platform for you and your friends to reach new heights.

5

THE SCIENCE OF ACROYOGA

If I have seen further, it is by standing on the shoulders of giants.
—SIR ISAAC NEWTON

This quote from one of the brightest minds of science offers the perfect analogy to AcroYoga. The scientific revolution changed the way we see the world and the way we experiment with life. For hundreds of years, thousands of scientists shared their insights and challenged their colleagues' insights to yield the current models that we agree upon today about the natural world. During this time as a species, our collective projection of reality began to shift from intuitive and feeling-based experience to one lived through the mind and its observations of the micro and macro.

There are two main methods scientists use to arrive at conclusions about the natural world. First, there are discoveries that start as ideas or theories. Once a theory is proposed it can be tested by doing different experiments, measuring

the results, and then either confirming or negating the theory. Einstein thought that light would be bent by the warping of space-time. Four years later, English astronomers Arthur Eddington and Frank Watson Dyson confirmed Einstein's general theory of relativity through experimentation. Second, there are discoveries based on observing what is happening in the world, and then attempting to explain what is observed. At the ripe old age of twenty-two, Charles Darwin dedicated five years of his life to traveling by boat to observe thousands of plants and animals. His studies led him to develop the theory of evolution and publish the book *The Origin of Species*.

AcroYoga is a blend of both methods. Jenny and I had a theory that our collective skills could be used to empower adults to play, yogis to become more acrobatic, and a global community to form around a physical practice that would make people better versions of themselves. After nearly twenty years of collecting empirical data and conducting countless experiments as a practitioner and teacher to thousands, I have synthesized AcroYoga in a scientific way that is easy to understand.

At the core of AcroYoga is the joy people feel doing it and the excitement people feel watching it. It takes the best of three ancient practices and fuses them in a way that dissolves perceived barriers as we relearn how to trust and play with one another. It is a practice that you can never fully master, because the better you get at it the more there is to learn.

When I first started traveling the world and meeting other acrobats, I realized that we all have different names for the same skills. The famous lift in the movie *Dirty Dancing* is called "front bird" by many acrobats. Dutch acrobats call it *snoek,* which is the name of a fish! If you are a high-level acrobat you can freestyle without language and have a fun acrobatic exchange, but if you wanted to do a specific skill with someone who speaks a different language, you would have to draw it with stick figures or mime

the skill with your body.

Over the course of my career, I have learned many different movement languages that informed the language of AcroYoga. It started with gymnastics, then sports acrobatics, cheerleading, and finally yoga. I had to invent new names and terms as the practice expanded. It was not easy to codify this infinitely complex practice, but I am so happy that after years of traveling, teaching, and sharing these terms, there are now millions of AcroYogis who share a common language and can all play together. Just as pilots around the world speak one international language, so AcroYogis can fly together because we speak the same language of flying poses.

The periodic table of elements, describing the building blocks of the universe, took many scientists over 100 years to piece together. This chart has unified how people on earth speak about the physical world, at least at the atomic level. I realized that if I truly wanted to reach one billion AcroYogis worldwide, we would need to be able to communicate on a foundational level that is at least as basic as hydrogen and oxygen. So I drew inspiration from the periodic chart to organize AcroYoga in a methodical and universal way.

All AcroYoga skills can be broken down into pure, individual elements that can then be combined into more complex compounds or skills. Many people live their lives without really understanding what's happening around them on an atomic level. The same is true for AcroYoga—many talented practitioners don't know the basic elements of the complex skills or poses that they perform. But no matter your training or level of practice, the AcroYoga Table of Elements will help you understand the complexity of AcroYoga by mapping it out in a way that helps you take your practice to higher levels of refinement and mastery.

I was super lucky to have a handful of masters who made me refine the shit out of the basics, which is how I became a world-class acrobat. I also had two injuries in my career that forced me to modify my training for many months and refine very simple, boring, and important skills even further. Putting attention to the right elements in your practice will greatly increase your potential. A high-level AcroYogi could do everything in the chart in a day. But realistically, this content can be studied and refined for a lifetime. The best in their sport all have a similar recipe

What "AcroYoga" means: *connection on the edge*
How we do it: in community—base, flyer, spotter
Why we do it: to support all people through movement, connection, and play

that begins with drilling the basics so they become second nature.

The AcroYoga Table of Elements includes the building blocks of the most important static poses of AcroYoga. The elements are organized from foundational at the bottom to more advanced at the top. The three colors correspond with the three roots of AcroYoga: red for solar acrobatic practices, blue for lunar therapeutic practices, and purple for yoga practices. Each pose has an abbreviation, a number, and a photo. There are ten different categories that contain poses designed to align, open, and strengthen the body. You can think of the elements in this table as the 94 ingredients you have to work with in the AcroYoga kitchen. I have prepared some soups, appetizers, and main courses out of these ingredients that you will get to taste later in the book.

THE ACROYOGA

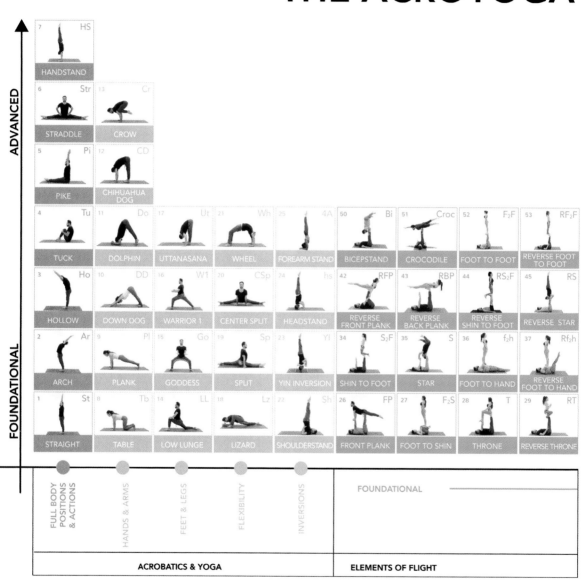

TABLE OF ELEMENTS

						94 FL FOLDED LEAF

63 Pr PRESENCE	69 Cp COMPASSION	75 Pe PEACE	81 BAT BAT	87 Sq SQUAT	93 Lo LOTUS
62 Cf CONFIDENCE	68 Tr TRUST	74 SK SELF KNOWLEDGE	80 BL BACK LEAF	86 Se SEIZA	92 Ea EASY POSE

54 BH₂H BABY HAND TO HAND	55 RBH₂H REVERSE BABY HAND TO HAND	56 h₂h HAND TO HAND	57 Rh₂h REVERSE HAND TO HAND	61 Cl CLARITY	67 Re RECEPTIVITY	73 Al ALIGNMENT	79 Wa WALNUT	85 He HERO POSE	91 Bu BUTTERFLY
46 TS TUCK SIT	47 RTS REVERSE TUCK SIT	48 Oss OUTSIDE STAR	49 ROss REVERSE OUTSIDE STAR	60 Co COMMUNICATION	66 Li LISTENING	72 Un UNDERSTANDING	78 RP REVERSE PRAYER	84 Mo MONKEY	90 Ja JANUSIRSASANA
38 SS SHOULDER STAND	39 RIss REVERSE INSIDE STAR	40 Iss INSIDE STAR	41 RSS REVERSE SHOULDER STAND	59 Fu FUN	65 Su SUPPORT	71 Cn CONNECTION	77 HFW HIGH FLYING WHALE	83 HK HALF KNEELING	89 Ch CHILDS POSE
30 BP BACK PLANK	31 BB BACK BIRD	32 SB STRADDLE BAT	33 RF₂S REVERSE FOOT TO SHIN	58 So SOLAR	64 Lu LUNAR	70 Ba BALANCE	76 LB LIFTED BUTTERFLY	82 HT HALF TABLE	88 Sv SAVASANA

	ADVANCED	ACROBATICS	THERAPEUTICS	YOGA	THERAPEUTIC FLYING	THAI STANCES	RECOVERY & MEDITATION POSES
	ELEMENTS OF FLIGHT	**NOBLE ELEMENTS**			**THERAPEUTICS & YOGA**		

ACROYOGA PRINCIPLES

1. Strangers Are Friends You Haven't Flown Yet.

We are taught in the modern world not to talk to strangers. I think this story needs an update. I have flown thousands of "strangers" for the first time, many of whom had a life-changing experience. We can extend friendship to all people, especially strangers. We have so much to gain by being nice to all people and assuming they are worthy of our kindness.

2. Community Begins with Three.

Base, flyer, and spotter form the smallest community. Everything that you learn in this group, especially when you get better at training higher-level and higher-risk skills, can support and enrich how you function in all the other communities you are a part of.

We are social animals that thrive when we feel connected and supported by a group of people. Excelling at being in groups has tremendous value and will continue to show you where you are strong and where you have room to grow.

3. True Success Is When Everyone Wins.

If a base is happy but their flyer is scared, that is not success. If a flyer is happy but the base is bored, that is also not success. When partners align their goals with the quality of practice they desire, that is the win-win that defines success.

4. Fly People Before You Negotiate.

This rule has made many situations in my life easier. If I want to buy a car, I fly the salesman. If I want to ask for the hand of a beautiful woman in marriage, I fly her father. If I want to teach at a local yoga studio, I fly the owner first.

Sharing our gifts and offering a deep essence-based connection with others, before we use our analytical minds to talk about numbers and other details, has great power and potential. To get this book deal I met with five different publishers. I offered to fly all of the editors I met with, but just one accepted my offer. Daniela Rapp was the only person in those meetings who felt the magic of AcroYoga firsthand, and she came back with the best offer.

These principles are not just fluffy ideas that sound good; they form the basis for how I live my life. I am sure many of them will help you find success and make friends along the way too.

6

THE ART OF ACROYOGA

How You Do Anything Is How You Do Everything

The Pyramids were built one stone at a time.
—YEVGENY MARCHENKO, COACH OF THE 2004 OLYMPIC GOLD MEDAL—WINNING
USA GYMNASTICS TEAM

In 1998 I had the honor and pleasure to train and live with Yevgeny Marchenko for a week. My acrobatic partner and I came with some ambitious goals, including attempting a skill that had never been attempted before. We had been training a double pike backflip from my hands back to my hands. Imagine a person doing a double backflip on a trampoline. Now imagine that I am the trampoline and my partner is standing on my hands. Yevgeny looked at the skill in the spotting belt and said in a thick Russian accent, "That is a very deadly skill." After he talked me and my partner off of the cliff, he offered us a pearl of wisdom that changed our outlook completely. Yevgeny's philosophy is super simple and effective: If you make a positive, successful attempt at a skill, you are adding a stone to your pyramid. If you make a negative, unsuccessful attempt at a skill, you are taking a stone away from your pyramid. With Yevgeny's philosophy we decided to redirect our aim from super crazy skills nobody had ever done before, to building our base of stones in order to reach high-level skills more slowly and steadily. As we did more basic skills with positive results, we fortified our foundation, our confidence, our timing, and our potential. If we failed at the skills we were attempting we would take a step back and find a way to add stones to our pyramid again. After each competitive season of gymnastics, my coaches would go back and drill me on my most basic skills to clean up my technique. We also did limitless amounts of very boring and painful strength and flexibility training. I didn't love it, but when I put those strength and flexibility gains on top of my newly refined and optimized technique, I had a higher level of mastery and a new baseline from which to keep growing.

One of the big lessons from those early training experiences that has stuck with me is that *how you do anything is how you do everything*. Giving the simple, foundational elements of a practice huge amounts of energy and attention is how you move toward more advanced skills. Similarly, if we want to achieve complex movements or "pinnacle" postures like handstand, we simply need to break them down into their component skills. Once you have mastered these building blocks, advanced postures and skills naturally begin to come within reach. This section of the book will offer you the tools to progressively build up your movement potential.

There are so many ways to live and what we do each day becomes our life's story. In the race to chase skills or titles or anything that creates the illusion of success, we can easily lose sight of how beautiful the journey of life can be. One definition of winning at life can be how

well we play it each day. I have been so blessed to train with masters and witness how masters train students in various disciplines. I believe and practice that it's a combination of discipline and freedom, thinking and feeling, that yields the best results in our practices and lives.

WHAT IS TRAINING?

Training is a systematic approach to building our skills in a given discipline. It usually includes the components of goal-setting and progress-tracking. It can be a blend of identifying our current strengths and weaknesses, then laying out a plan to enhance our abilities and refine our technique. Smart training can get you results faster and more safely, and help you develop aspects of your practice that bring more richness to your life. It can also build strong relationships with others that train in the same disciplines.

"Technique" can be described as the methods we use to do something. It is how we use what we have, ideally with increasing precision and efficiency. In movement and sports, technique can be seen as the ability to maximize the two inputs of strength and flexibility.

In AcroYoga there are many ways to train technique, but the outcome isn't judged by human beings—it is rewarded or punished by gravity. The better the technique, the more repetitions can be done, the longer static postures can be maintained, and the higher skills can be reached.

Body control is also key to improving technique. When doing a push-up, nothing in the body should move other than the arms extending and bending. When the head is moving, and the spine is dancing, and the feet are coming apart and together, technical efficiency is very low. If an athlete overcompensates for inefficient technique with massive amounts of strength, their actions can be more destructive to their practice than beneficial. Clean and efficient technique is paramount.

Overall, smart training is an art and a science, a feeling and a knowing. In the scientific sense, training provides very clear frameworks, measurements, and progressions. It can get you further with less effort. It can be a container that satiates the mind with structure so the body can learn without the mind wondering what to do next. Training is a great place to go deeper in understanding where you are strong and where you still have potential for growth. It provides a systematic building of trust in relating to partners, coaches, and others you train around.

As methodical as training can be, it can also be deeply informed by artistry and creativity. Are you able to express your emotion through your practice? Can you find a way for your life's dreams to be a part of your physical practice? Are you brave enough to express your vulnerability in your practice? These are some of the paintbrushes that are available to us to soften the edges of science. Movement is like a blank canvas that you can fill in with your feelings; this is how you can invite more artistry into your practice.

HOW IS SUCCESS IN TRAINING MEASURED?

Success depends on the definition of your end goal. If you want to get a handstand, you have to define what that means. "I want to not be afraid of attempting a handstand by myself," or "I want to be able to hold a handstand for ten seconds," are measurable goals. Saying, "I want to get a handstand," is not. Once your goals are clearly defined you can set up metrics to gauge and quantify your progress.

If your goals are skill-based, you can work backwards from your end goal. In the beginning stages of reaching your movement goals you might not have enough context to build a progressive plan to get there. Good news! There are thousands of certified AcroYoga teachers and thousands more gymnastics coaches around the world, so building a solid training plan with professional support to maximize your efforts is accessible almost anywhere.

Strength and flexibility goals are also very important parts of your training. Quantifying how many repetitions you can do in strength exercises or how long you can hold static poses are effective measurements of strength. Flexibility can be measured by how much range of motion you have in any one direction with your body. This range is not only measured by centimeters but also by ease. Ease comes when your strength and flexibility are balanced, compatible, and complementary.

GOAL SETTING

To get anywhere in a discipline you must clarify another triad—'what,' 'how,' and 'why.' Learning to define these things will help you be more strategic in developing your practice. These three checkpoints are also very important in how you build your practice with others. The more clear and aligned you are here with your partner, the more ease you will have in how you train and how you assess the success of your training.

The 'what' speaks to defining the name or description of the skill or goal. This is usually the easiest of the three to identify, and it is key for organizing your training and communicating with others. Your 'what' can be, "I will do three sets of push-ups after three sets of planks."

'How' speaks to the method or technique used to train the skill. I hope the following sentence sticks with you: *Your body trains your mind and your mind trains your body.* Your mind, left to its own devices, can drive you crazy, especially if you do not let the wisdom of the body affect your decisions, your training, and your life. The body is easier to understand—you just have to listen. It speaks in feelings and sensations and says, "I like" or "I don't like." There are layers, of course, to each. Your body might not like the last few repetitions of strength training, but the feeling after is pure bliss. When the body is performing at a high level the mind takes a back seat, and this changing of the guard is vital to how you train for any sport. When you are in a static pose, be it a handstand or seated meditation, your body becomes a container for a clarifying fire to quiet your mind. If your mind wavers, peace and harmony are lost. The stillness of the body can train the mind and vice versa.

The 'why' is your motivation for getting off the couch to do the skill. Until you know your 'why' you cannot clearly know your 'how.' There is no way to determine if your training methods are correct until you decide where you want to go with your practice. Is arching your back in a handstand wrong? Many would say yes, but if you want to do a scorpion handstand and put your feet on your head, arching is the way to that goal. Your 'why' can also be a desired effect of your training. For example, "I want to do AcroYoga to become more confident," or "I want to do AcroYoga to be able to help others feel empowered."

Your 'why' is what moves you at the deepest level. It is your spiritual connection to your actions—your soul food, your mission statement, your reason for being. It's the part that is greater than you and the bigger the goal the more magical, mystical, spiritual energy

you will need to harness to get you to your desired outcome. When we lack clarity, we often struggle with a lack of motivation or will. As you come to know your 'why,' you can dedicate yourself more deeply and come much closer to mastery than if you do things for unclear reasons.

TRAINING PITFALLS

Training has the potential to take the joy out of a practice and cause injury if it is too intense and not balanced with recovery. When you go deep with one partner, your focus can become so narrow and your practice so exclusive that your wisdom is not shared with the community. Jamming is the opposite of training. AcroYoga jams are creative gatherings similar to music jams where there is a variable amount of structure and a large amount of in-the-moment, unpredictable collaboration. If training is to refine, jamming is to discover. There are always new skills, variations, and ways of doing life. The more you train the fewer surprises there will be in your practice, and if you overtrain you might miss these gems.

WHAT IS MASTERY?

All technique is to be forgotten and the unconscious to be left alone to handle the situation. Technique will assert its wonders automatically or spontaneously. To float in totality, to have no technique, is to have all technique.
—BRUCE LEE

Easier said than done, Bruce! I understand by experiencing it myself what it feels like to train a drill for years and then in some mystical moment, maybe after ten thousand hours of doing the skill, the mind, body, and spirit converge and a flow state is achieved. The impossible becomes easy, and the struggle is only in realizing that you can do anything you dedicate your whole being to.

The word *discipline* comes from the word "disciple." To master something you have to dedicate yourself to it and usually become a disciple to a teacher or a method. I am often impressed by the impatience of students. Arno L'Hermitte is an osteopath from France and one of the founders of the Thai Circus in Laos. He is brilliant in his approach to teaching principles of touch. He can teach many things, but only if the student has put in the time to master the basics. The basics of touch and

healing are simple and at the same time deeply nuanced. When he teaches palming he will often say, "Be humble and repeat." Humility and repetition are very related and are a huge part of the mastery of any practice. After spending a year on basics, a student could learn more advanced material in one day than in five years of only chasing the flashy tricks.

I trained handstands and one-arm handstands with a Chinese circus master named Lu Yi for about five years off and on. We did the same exercises every session. The expansion was not in doing harder or fancier moves; it was in being connected to every little thing happening in my body while doing the same poses again and again. Gymnasts are some of the most highly trained athletes on the planet. Usually they get no more than one week off per year. When they return from their vacation they go back to basics. They start at the foundation and build everything back up with renewed attention to detail. An advanced athlete can repeatedly do basic skills with advanced awareness, whereas many intermediate athletes often pursue the next shiny goal as soon as they can survive a skill. Yoga masters don't stop doing sun salutations, a very "easy" set of traditional yoga postures, even after decades of practice.

Each person has preferred ways to learn based on their own nature. In my decades of training I have found many patterns and techniques that have helped me and countless students I have worked with. Here I share with you those insights.

KEYS TO MASTERY

» Find teachers you trust who have experience you do not.
» Be selective in who you dedicate yourself to as a student, as your teachers will have the potential to steer you and your life to an immense degree.
» Have a beginner's mind. If your cup is empty, you have the potential to fully receive what any person or experience has to offer you.
» Resist filtering information initially. Oftentimes new information feels foreign. Even if it does not make sense, try to absorb it at first. If you filter everything on the way in, you might miss something that could change your life.
» Take time to digest and revisit what you learn, especially things that do not make sense to you.
» If after some time there are still things you do not understand, go back to the teacher and present your questions.

Any masterful teacher shows you aspects of yourself you do not see yet. They guide you to a new place of understanding; they are not magicians who make miracles happen for you. Digest and integrate the information from your teachers and you will find your own wellspring of wisdom.

"The ancient masters were profound and subtle.
Their wisdom was unfathomable.
There is no way to describe it;
all we can describe is their appearance.

They were careful as someone crossing an iced-over stream.
Alert as a warrior in enemy territory.
Courteous as a guest.
Fluid as melting ice.
Shapable as a block of wood.
Receptive as a valley.
Clear as a glass of water.

Do you have the patience to wait till your mud settles
and the water is clear?
Can you remain unmoving till the right action
arises by itself?

The master doesn't seek fulfillment.
Not seeking, not expecting,
she is present, and can welcome all things."

—LAO TZU

NOBLE ELEMENTS OF TRAINING

These Noble Elements are key to unlocking your training techniques. AcroYoga is one playground where you can train your body, mind, and relationships. The wisdom you collect in this practice and the methods that you learn as you train can be applied to other aspects of your life. When you are training well you will know clearly what you want, using receptivity to find more ease and eventually optimal alignment.

Clarity (Cl)

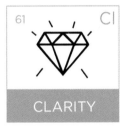

Clarity takes the cloud of the unknown and distills it into something known. An eagle, with its keen eyesight, razor-like beak, and mighty talons could be the totem animal of clarity. It is sharp, focused, and direct. Clarity increases as you move from scattered to focused.

I chose a diamond to represent this element because diamonds are the hardest substance on earth and they are formed under huge amounts of pressure and heat. Under these conditions we too can clarify like a diamond.

Receptivity (Re)

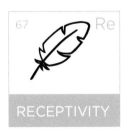

Receptivity is the soft feather that can polish the diamond. Its strength is in gentleness and the ability to realign. Moving from a place of rigidity to openness increases your receptivity.

A butterfly could be the totem animals of receptivity. In a windstorm this clever insect can angle and flap its beautiful wings in just the right ways to let the wind take it wherever it wants to go. Receptivity is a core element of acrobatics, yoga, and healing, and as it increases, a new depth of practice is possible and more ease can be found. This journey into being more and more receptive will allow for harder and more elegant variations in your AcroYoga practice.

Alignment (Al)

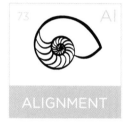

The nautilus is one of many expressions of life that contains predictable mathematical relationships based on the golden ratio. The golden ratio is found all throughout nature because it maximizes structural integrity and support. We all are made of different-shaped bones and muscles and there is not one way to align for all people and all things, but there is a golden ratio inherent in our design, and becoming familiar with it can be hugely beneficial.

Alignment can be in relation to our bones, to the way a partner wants to be interacted with, or to the environment around us. When things are not aligned there is struggle. The simple and profound practice of aligning our thoughts, words, and actions can help us struggle less with life. If we pay attention to the many interactions we have each day, we can become aware of where we are aligned and misaligned with those around us.

Alignment is the result of practicing with clarity and receptivity. When things are properly aligned there is a quality of ease and flow. This is true in a Front Plank (FP), in your relationships, and in your life.

SMART TRAINING PRINCIPLES

1. Little Details Are Not Little.

Handstands are one of the more difficult poses students regularly attempt. It is a supernatural expression of a super complex system, so to have success you have to start from the ground and work your way up, one set of bones and muscles at a time.

   The way I train and teach is rooted in the little details because the little details are what will support or limit your progress as an AcroYogi. Remember, after spending a year on basics, you could learn more advanced material in one day than in five years of only chasing the flashy tricks.

2. The First Three Don't Count.

The mind can be like a puppy; it craves attention, has lots of energy, and can be overly enthusiastic. Often acrobats will attempt something for the first time, then spend many minutes debating what went right and wrong. All of this time spent debating is less valuable than getting in a few more attempts and then seeing if there is a trend.

   It's not that you can't learn from your first attempt, and safety conversations can definitely be supportive. But don't get so invested in theories until you have three attempts to analyze.

3. Make New Mistakes.

Being mindful of each attempt and being able to modify small things about how you are doing a skill is how you improve your ability to do AcroYoga.

If you attempt a skill repeatedly and have the same negative result, you will make bad habits stronger. A classic example is attempting to kick up to a handstand: attempt one—*not enough power*; attempt two—*not enough power*; attempts three through ten—*same result*.

If you make the same mistake three times in a row you should change your approach: usually that means doing something easier and building a technical skill or confidence in yourself. While practicing each skill, you can and should pause, evaluate, and decide if something needs to change. New mistakes are golden, and as scary as they can be, seek them out.

4. More Advanced Means More Versatile.

I believe if you are truly advanced you can have success in AcroYoga with anyone.

I have had students come up to me at acrobatic trainings to request a new partner because they felt they were more advanced than their partner. I usually respond with the mantra above.

They don't like to hear that because their sense of satisfaction is dependant on how quickly they can learn advanced tricks. The truth is, a less advanced partner can greatly further your practice because they demand higher levels of listening, support, and clarity in your communication and movement.

SOLO SMART TRAINING PRACTICE

Card Throwing Exercise

For this exercise all you need is a deck of cards, something to throw the cards into (a hat, bucket, bowl, etc.), and fifteen minutes. This game is easy and effective in helping you learn how to develop theories for improving a skill.

With a single deck of cards you have fifty-two attempts to see how many you can throw into the target. Choose your distance from the target, and if you get more than half the cards into the target on your first round, make your target smaller or your distance bigger.

Take a few practice rounds to find the combination of distance and target size that allows you to get about ten cards in the target. From there, keep the distance and target the same and try three more rounds. Work on your foundation—how you are standing and how you hold the card, and your actions—how much you flick your wrist, the extension of your arm, swinging versus punching, etc.

How many cards are you able to throw into the target after your practice rounds?

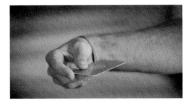

BEGINNER: 5–15 cards

INTERMEDIATE: 16–26 cards

ADVANCED: 27–45 cards

EXPERT: 46–52 cards

As soon as you master your dominant hand, humbly start the process on your other hand. Or for advanced students, throw the cards with your eyes closed!

PARTNER SMART TRAINING PRACTICE

Coaching Plank ATB: Alignment, Tightness, Balance

Alignment in theory is easy—straight is strong and bones are where we start when aligning the body. Once your bones are in a vertical, straight alignment you can involve your muscles to squeeze onto the bone layer.

When the bones are aligned and the muscles activated around this alignment, you have the most basic and important part of acrobatics figured out—bone stacking.

This exercise teaches you how to find a vertical arm line and how to engage all of your muscles. Once you feel this on the ground, it will show you what you need to do when you fly Front Plank (FP).

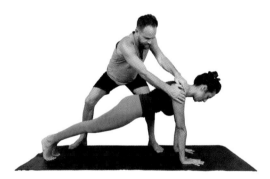

The following is a two-person drill: one person does the skill while the other coaches. Both base and flyer are supported by doing this exercise.

ALIGNMENT:

» Begin with hands shoulder width apart, middle fingers parallel to each other, **arms vertical and straight**. Feet together, head neutral, spine straight.

» After looking at their friend's alignment, the coach **communicates what can be improved**.

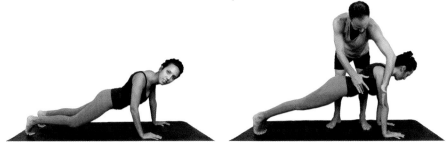

Misaligned Plank   Aligned Plank

TIGHTNESS:

» The coach gently **pushes different parts of the body** to wake up and activate the muscles until the whole body is stiff, unified, and engaged.

» Your goal as the coach is to **help your friend find muscular integrity** and fire all the muscles they have to hold their plank shape. You can do too much, but you can also do too little.

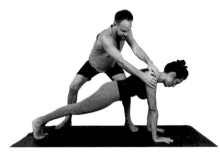
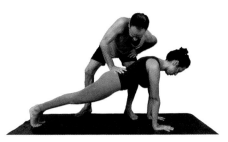

Test Arm Tightness   Test Core Tightness

BALANCE:

» Once the bones are aligned and the muscles tightened, the final step is balance. As the student, **lift one foot or one hand off the ground**.

» This can be done in Table (Ta) pose (knees on the ground) for more stability. If that is easy, try lifting one hand and the opposite foot off the ground.

» As the coach, help your friend keep their planted **arm vertical and body engaged**—alignment and tightness always help balance.

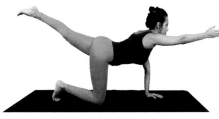

Table Balance Drill

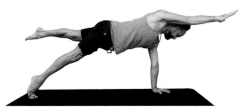

Plank Balance Drill

VISIT **WWW.ACROYOGA.ORG/MCP** TO DOWNLOAD A FREE WORKBOOK, WATCH TUTORIALS, AND FIND OUR COMPANION VIDEO COURSE TO HELP YOU ACTIVATE THE PRINCIPLES AND PRACTICES DISCUSSED IN THIS CHAPTER.

7

STRENGTH TRAINING

You have power over your mind—not outside events. Realize this, and you will find strength.
—MARCUS AURELIUS

I remember very clearly from a young age wanting to have a six-pack and huge biceps. As a child I learned that having big muscles was attractive to women and gained instant respect from other men. When I started training gymnastics, I was not especially strong. Within my first three months I was able to do all the variations of splits thanks to my natural flexibility, but strength was another animal. Because of this my coaches made me do lots of strength training. I did not care much for it—I wanted to play on the trampoline and do acrobatics with my partner David.

By the time I made the competitive team, our coach had us warming up with pull-ups, push-ups, bar dips, V-ups, and running stairs—one hundred of each. I don't think I ever managed to do one hundred pull-ups in a practice, but I got used to doing high repetitions of strength training exercises before every gymnastics session. Once I got to my first competition, I could see the clear advantages of this approach: Because of our strength we could do the bonus moves that granted us a higher base score. We could hold the static poses without shaking. My passion for competing and being able to do higher-level gymnastics and acrobatics became my motivation for strength training.

I still do not have a six-pack or huge biceps, but I learned where my motivation for building strength comes from, and I regularly dip back into my emotions and desires to keep me coming back to the very boring, not at all sexy, but hugely beneficial practice of strength training. How we look does not define our strength. Strength starts in the mind and is reinforced by skillful, progressive training to improve the efficiency of the power we already have.

WHAT IS PHYSICAL STRENGTH?

Strength is a measure of how much power, stability, or endurance one has. There are many ways to define and expand on these qualities. When talking about strength, it is helpful to recognize the tissues through which our strength is exerted—the muscles, fascia, tendons, ligaments, bones, and at the root of it all, the mind. If we think we are strong, we will be strong; if we think we are weak, we will be weak. Our thoughts create our reality. We will always be gaining or losing strength over time depending on our practices, but our attitudes have an even bigger impact.

Muscles are the most obvious physical parts of us that make us strong, and they are supported or limited by many other aspects of our anatomy. Our bones are the hardest, and one could say the strongest parts of our body. Ligaments are the network that keep our bones aligned and together. Tendons connect our muscles to our bones. Fascia can be understood as the "web" that holds our watery bits together. If you think of an orange, all the stringy white parts are like the fascia. Without fascia we would be a bloody mess; the elasticity of this tissue works with

our muscles to create the spring in our step. Much of what generates strength is knowing how to leverage the advantages of each tissue for different tasks you are asking your body to perform.

Our muscles have evolved different mechanisms for working in the presence or absence of oxygen. Acrobatics is more of an *anaerobic* discipline, where we do short bursts of high-intensity work. *Aerobic* disciplines, on the other hand, require the steady and continual burning of oxygen as activities are performed. There are two types of muscle tissue, called fast twitch and slow twitch, that support these different types of movement. A sprinter has more fast-twitch muscles, and a marathon runner has more slow-twitch muscles.

Dynamic strength is the exertion of force through movement while static strength is the ability to hold shapes for longer and longer periods of time, such as how long you can hang from a bar or do a handstand. Static strength rests upon the alignment of the bones and the levels of muscular integration and mental steadiness. The more calm the mind and the more clear the willpower, the longer static holds can be. Dynamic power increases by controlling the order and timing of how muscles fire. Olympic weightlifters are the masters of this art. AcroYogis train the same types of elements, as gravity truly teaches us to time and execute our dynamic power.

No matter what kind of training you do there is a recipe for maximizing the effort you invest to build the right kind of strength. The stronger you are, the more potential you have to move your body and to move other objects. Strength can give you stability and the power to keep yourself grounded and not be moved by others. Being strong can also keep you from being injured if you fall. A strong body will be able to take more of a beating without getting beat. If you're thinking, "Okay, yes, I want to be stronger," our next step is quantifying strength.

HOW STRENGTH IS MEASURED

Speed

This is easy enough to understand—speed is a measure of how fast you can go or how many repetitions of an action you can do in a set amount of time. Newton's second law ($F=mA$) shows us that speed is a great way to gauge our dynamic strength. With a fixed mass like your body, the force you generate is greater if you do things faster.

Load and Volume

This is represented by the quantity of repetitions you can do with a fixed amount of weight, as long as quality of technique does not suffer. *Work = force x distance*: the more distance, or reps, the more work and the more of a workout you are getting.

Endurance

Endurance is defined by how long you can endure or sustain an activity. Static holds for duration are a practice in endurance and they train the mind and the muscles to stay in integrity under stress.

Personal Best

Personal best is defined by the maximum weight you can lift in a certain exercise, how long you can hold a certain pose, or how many repetitions of an exercise you can do in a row. Timing your handstands or increasing your push-up count are examples of testing and training your personal best.

TYPES OF STRENGTH TRAINING

Inherently, every student has different goals, strengths, and areas of potential growth. With the help of a coach or trainer you can build your strength in specific ways that will help you reach your goals. Below are some of the items on the strength-building menu:

Resistance Training

Resistance training is a form of exercise that improves muscular stamina and control. During a resistance training workout, you move your limbs against resistance provided by your bodyweight, a partner's bodyweight, bands, kettlebells, weighted bars, or dumbbells.

Olympic Weightlifting

Olympic weightlifting is a sport in which the athlete attempts a maximum-weight single lift of a barbell loaded with weight plates. There are many similarities between standing acrobatics and Olympic weight-lifting. Many CrossFit athletes thrive in standing acrobatics due to this training.

Calisthenics

Calisthenics derives from the joining of the Greek words *kalos,* meaning "beautiful," and *sthenos,* meaning "strength." The word was originally used to refer to exercises done by young women, but it later gained the more general meaning that we now know: bodyweight exercises performed without special equipment that develop strength. This includes push-ups, jumping jacks, mountain climbers, burpees, etc.

Tightness Drills

Tightness drills are designed to get a group of muscles to fire isometrically in a particular region of the body. Isometric squeezing is the contracting of muscles not to create movement, but rather to create tightness and unification in the body. Sometimes they are full-body drills, and other times they focus on one specific part of the body. This is a mind-connecting-to-muscles kind of training. It will not make your muscles huge, but you will learn to unify your body to become strong and steady like a tree.

Partner Acrobatics

In partner acrobatics, our friends become our equipment as we train different ways to use a person's bodyweight for building balance, strength, and flexiblity. Because the "weight" is a living, breathing, *moving* human being, these practices are very effective ways to improve stabilization, communication, and listening. Partner acrobatics includes L-base training, counterbalances, and standing acrobatics, and they are all excellent full-body strength training activities, especially if you base and fly. The skills you learn in these practices result in better and smarter means to building both physical strength and human relationships.

HOW TO BUILD STRENGTH

Proper Technique Wins

Knowing your foundations and actions helps you understand what should and shouldn't move in a given exercise. Easy variations and clean technique with lower reps are good ways to start so that you learn to move force through your body clearly and efficiently. You are building good habits more than just muscles.

Max-In versus Max-Out

Most people know and dread max-outs. This is when you do a static hold or repetitions of a skill until you fail. What is great about max-out training is that it pushes your limits, helping you to develop new physical and mental strengths. The price you pay when doing max-outs is that your form and technique almost always suffer. By contrast, "max-in" is short for maximum integrity. This is where you go for as long as you can with clean form, and then exit with dignity. What this really speaks to is how well you are

aligned, because proper alignment creates ease for longer holds or more reps. With static holds like handstands, you can also incorporate counting your breaths to add a layer of calm.

Especially when doing partner acrobatic strength training, integrity and form are key to building your ideal practice. Our training patterns create our habits, so how you do each push-up either advances your practice or erodes it. For this reason, max-ins are a smarter approach to training than max-outs.

Range of Motion (ROM)

You are only as strong as your weakest link. In acrobatics and gymnastics, the reality is that you need strength in your full range of flexibility. If you do push-ups in a very narrow range of motion, it will show as soon as you get a partner on top of your hands. The weight of their body will push your arms past the point you normally train in, and you will get stuck. For this reason, we emphasize building strength in the full range of motion available to our bodies.

Variations

There are always ways to increase the inclusivity and intensity of strength elements in your training. Changing the angle of the arms, the amplitude of the range of motion, adding or removing points of contact with the floor, jumping off the floor, doing more or fewer reps, holding statically for more or less time— these are all great ways to add variability and resilience to your practice. For example, if you are good at squats, do squat jumps, or squats on one foot, or with a partner on your back.

Increase Speed

For strength training that has dynamic movement, faster is better as long as you don't lose clean technique. Here again $F=mA$ proves the value of acceleration. Faster means more force, and more force means more acrobatic potential. Think of speed like the chili pepper of your movement practice. Chili is only appreciated if present in the right amount in the right dish, so use it only when your technique can support it. Fast sloppy movements are like hot sauce on vanilla ice cream. Not needed, not appreciated.

STRENGTH TRAINING PITFALLS

There are people who love the aesthetic of big muscles and train to get them. But if huge muscles are built without flexibility the body becomes a time bomb. Huge forces exerted on tight, tense tissues can cause serious injuries. There can also be a tendency to train one movement so much that you build up repetitive stress injuries. People confuse the importance of the number of reps with the quality of reps when strength training. Remember, you are building acrobatic patterns through strength training, and muscle size is secondary.

STRENGTH TRAINING PRINCIPLES

1. Be Consistent.

If you had two choices to build strength—a weekend boot camp with Arnold Schwarzenegger or you in your garage for fifteen minutes a day doing simple bodyweight exercises, which would you pick? Of course you would choose the first option—I have always wanted to meet the Governator too!

Many people think they don't have enough time during the week to strength train. When you are a weekend warrior you might feel a lot of sensation in sore muscles as your body sends out war cries during your last set. But in all fairness you are not really building strength the easy way.

Every night when you sleep you have an army of little helpers repairing and rejuvenating the cells in your body. Doing little bits of training and then getting the proper rest is a much better recipe for big and consistent gains in strength than weekend boot camp training. Being consistent means dedicating time to certain strength training exercises for months or even years.

2. Receptive Before Strong.

There are few things more powerful than lava. Measuring between 700 and 1200 degrees Celsius, it is one of the hottest and strongest forces on planet Earth. Lava tubes created by the cooling of the lava in some areas help to direct the flow of hotter, more molten lava. It is this cooling lunar energy that, when applied before the blast of hot solar energy, helps guide the fire to the right place. Within true power lies receptivity.

When you are basing anything, be soft to invite your flyer into the collaboration, then strong to reinforce the trust you are offering. As a flyer, softness is taking a moment to let go of control and find your base's points of contact.

If you are strong before receptive, collaboration with your partner will feel more demanding than inviting. As a general rule, think lunar then solar, feminine then masculine, receptive then strong.

3. The Mind is the Strongest Muscle.

Technically the mind is not a muscle, but it is the origin of our physical strength and weakness. If you think you can't do something, you will be right. If you think you can do something, you are at least moving in the right direction.

It costs nothing to believe that things are possible. I had wanted to do a one-arm handstand since the first time I saw the skill in the movie *Star Wars* when I was five years old. I believed in the Force and in my capabilities. Twenty-three years later I met Master Lu Yi, the Chinese circus Yoda, and boom—I got my one-arm handstand.

The cost of believing in your dreams is zero; the cost of not believing in them is immeasurable. Part III will give you much more to work with on this subject.

SOLO STRENGTH PRACTICE

Push-ups

This is one of the best overall dynamic strength-building calisthenic exercises! It correlates to both flyers and bases finding ease in AcroYoga. This upper-body focused drill can also teach full-body integration, especially if you squeeze your feet together the whole time.

If you're new to push-ups, focus on keeping your core engaged to maintain a neutral spine. At all levels, remember to train in your full range of motion, which in this case means bending your arms as far as you can. Ultimately, you want to kiss the floor with your nose on the way down without compromising the integrity of your form.

FOUNDATION:

» Start lying down on your belly, arms bent, hands on the ground a bit by your ribs, wider than shoulder width apart, with your fingers spread wide and middle fingers parallel to each other.

» Whatever variation you choose, keep your legs, knees, and feet squeezed together and engage your abdomen.

ACTIONS:

» Bend and extend the arms. This is the only visible action.

» The secondary action is squeezing your entire body.

BEGINNER: Knee Push-ups

» Bend your knees and place them on the ground, keeping your legs and feet together.

» Straighten and bend your arms, elbows wider than the hands as you bend them.

» Keep your body engaged and in a straight line from your head to your knees.

3 repetitions.

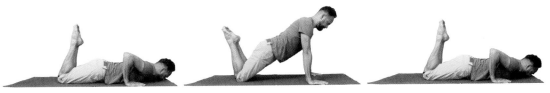

Knee Push-up Foundation   Arms Straighten   Arms Bend

INTERMEDIATE: Plank Push-ups

» Keep feet together and legs straight.

» Straighten and bend the arms, elbows wider than the hands as you bend them.

» Keep your body engaged and in a straight line from your head to your toes.

5 repetitions.

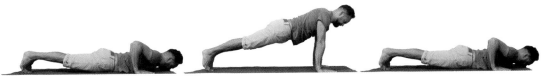

Plank Push-up Foundation   Arms Straighten   Arms Bend

ADVANCED: Jumping Knee Push-ups

» Bend knees and keep feet together. Straighten and bend the arms with explosive power, jumping off your hands, elbows wider than the hands as you bend them.

» Keep your body engaged and in a straight line from your head to your knees.

15 repetitions.

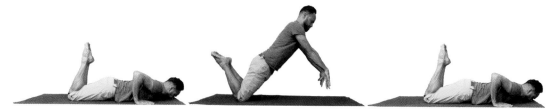

Knee Push-up with Jump Foundation   Jump with Full Extension   Arms Bend

EXPERT: Jumping Plank Push-ups

» Keep feet together and legs straight.

» Straighten and bend the arms with explosive power, jumping off your hands, elbows wider than the hands as you bend them.

» Keep your body engaged and in a straight line from your head to your toes.

15 repetitions.

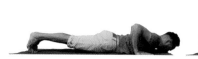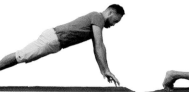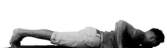

Plank Push-up with Jump Foundation   Jump with Full Extension   Arms Bend

PARTNER STRENGTH PRACTICE

Plank on Plank

The base makes a plank with their feet shoulder width of the flyer. The flyer holds the base's ankles, lifts their pointed foot to the top of the base's shoulder, then places the second foot on the base's other shoulder so that their plank is stacked directly on top of the base's plank.

BEGINNER:
10-second hold

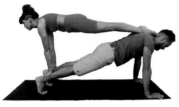

Hold Plank on Plank

INTERMEDIATE: 5-second hold, flyer does a push-up; 5-second hold, base does a push-up. Both at least half Range of Motion (ROM). *3 repetitions.*

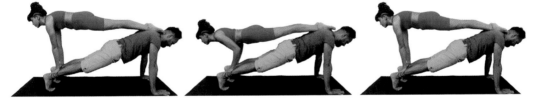

| Plank on Plank | Flyer Bends Arms | Flyer Straightens Arms |

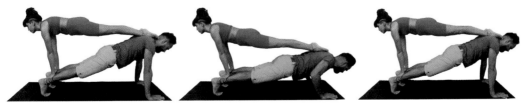

| Plank on Plank | Base Bends Arms | Base Straightens Arms |

ADVANCED:

5-second hold, flyer and base do a push-up at the same time.
Both half Range of Motion (ROM). *5 repetitions.*

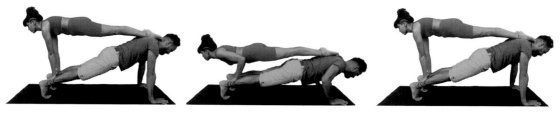

Plank on Plank   Both Bend Arms   Both Straighten Arms
                        Half (ROM)

EXPERT:

5-second hold, flyer and base do a push-up at the same time.
Both full Range of Motion (ROM). *10 repetitions.*

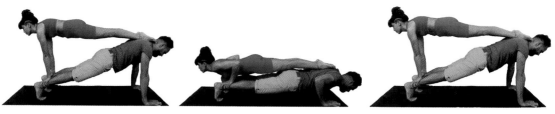
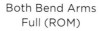

Plank on Plank   Both Bend Arms   Both Straighten Arms
                        Full (ROM)

VISIT *WWW.ACROYOGA.ORG/MCP* TO DOWNLOAD A FREE WORKBOOK, WATCH
TUTORIALS, AND FIND OUR COMPANION VIDEO COURSE TO HELP YOU ACTIVATE
THE PRINCIPLES AND PRACTICES DISCUSSED IN THIS CHAPTER.

REFLECT & BUILD YOUR STRENGTH

Strength Journaling is a practice that can unite the power of the mind with the strength of the body. As a result of examining our strengths, weaknesses, and desires, we can find natural intelligence in our training. This prompt is designed to uncover your potential and ignite inspiration unique to you.

Outward Reflection
1. Write the name of someone you know who you think is very strong.
2. What qualities does this "strong" person have?

Inward Reflection
3. Where do I have strength and power in my life?
4. Where in my life do I want more strength or power?
5. What habit, practice, or quality would support the strength of my relationships?

Make a Path Forward
6. What would success look like in my strength-building practice?
7. What skill or move would be a huge milestone for my expression of strength?
8. In pursuit of my strength goals, what exercises will I dedicate to? For how long?

As an example, your Strength Journaling might look something like this:
1. *Baya.*
2. *She is solid, fiery, and able to do just about anything she decides to do...*
3. *I am strong in my commitment to my morning practices. I have a lot of power in my legs, and my mind is strong in many ways.*
4. *I want more strength to ask for what I want/need from my friends. I also want more pulling strength.*
5. *Having fewer friends and giving more to those I really want to grow with would help strengthen my relationships.*
6. *Success would look like being able to climb harder routes at the climbing gym.*
7. *A huge milestone for me would be doing over 10 pull-ups in a row.*
8. *For the next month I will do 3 sets of pull-ups for two days on, one day off. I will also climb at the gym 2-3 times/week. For my internal strength I will practice voicing my needs. For my relationships I will call my closest friends once a week.*

8

FLEXIBILITY TRAINING

Body not stiff, mind stiff.
—SRI K. PATTABHI JOIS

As a gymnast and acrobat, I was always flexible and had to work more on strength to achieve my goals. By the time I retired from competitive sports acrobatics at twenty-three, I felt very accomplished in my career, but I knew there was still a lot more for me to explore. I thought I would finish college to satisfy my parents, then join Cirque du Soleil and eventually get back into competitive form to compete in the Olympics, once acrobatics became an Olympic sport.

At the time this seemed like a great plan (like many plans do!) but life threw me a curveball. I went to my first yoga class during my senior year of college and quickly learned a bunch of new ways in which I was not flexible at all! Lotus and pigeon were impossible for me, and there were all of these weird balance poses that served me one slice of humble pie after another. I got hooked on yoga right away and dedicated myself to becoming the most flexible human on earth. My teacher, Dharma Mittra, is famous for a poster with 908 poses that he has mastered. I saw this as my "homework," and got on my yoga mat daily to learn the ways of this mystical practice. Unfortunately, my enthusiasm won me a whole host of new injuries. I tore a meniscus in my knee forcing my legs into lotus. I hurt my shoulders bouncing in a hyper-extended downward dog pose. These injuries were the result of the inflexibility of my mind imposing its will on my body.

At the same time I was learning about healing arts, so healing those injuries was an instrumental part of my path. I was in a period in my life of experiencing the most change I had ever known. All of these shifts started in my mind, and from there the ideas slowly took root in my body. At the peak of my yoga phase, I was doing three to five hours of yoga per day, eating raw vegan food, and walking very slowly around New York City as a mindfulness practice. My dynamic acrobatic strength got converted into super bendy yogic flexibility over this period of time. I appeared in *Yoga Journal* magazine several times demonstrating the "correct" form in many difficult postures.

From there AcroYoga started gaining momentum and I came back to my first true love of acrobatics, resumed training more skills that built my strength, and went back to eating meat. These shifts over time reduced my flexibility. I did not realize how much of it I had lost until I was teaching at a yoga conference in Hong Kong in 2013 where my teacher Dharma Mitra was teaching as well. I took his class and was shocked by how many poses I could not do anymore. Thanks to all the yoga philosophy I had gained, I was not upset or attached to how my practice used to be, but I knew that if I wanted to regain flexibility I would have to shift my training, eating, and recovery practices. And that is exactly what I did.

In the life of my practice I have already climbed many mountains and reached many goals that have drastically shifted my body. I have also slipped back into the valleys of weakness, stiffness and inactivity. There is a benefit and cost to every decision you make in your training. Wherever you are, enjoy it, and know you can shift it over time. Life will offer you many opportunities where you get to reshape your patterns. Every time you do, you get to build your body back up, learning from what you have done well and not well. Growing your flexibility improves your movement potential, and also allows for greater efficiency in other skills you do. My hope is that the tools in this book can help you reach your goals *and* make new ones.

In the holy trinity of ATB, or alignment, tightness, and balance, your flexibility allows for you to find more ease aligning your bones in postures. You will learn more about this in Chapter 14, *Inversions and Coaching*. You need less strength when your motion is more fluid and there are fewer points of resistance in your body.

We are born mobile and flexible. Rigidity is a learned and earned quality that develops based on how we think, speak, and move. Our bodies actually change from around 80 percent to 70 percent water over our lifetimes. As we grow older we tend to lose mobility and literally harden from the inside out. But it doesn't have to be this way! Flexibility of mind, body, and spirit can be available to us at any age with proper training.

WHAT IS FLEXIBILITY?

Physically, flexibility is the ability to bend your body without breaking it. There are many fancy terms in the study of biomechanics to describe movement. No matter the term or part of the body, flexibility is one of the most important and underutilized aspects of movement training.

The ability to actively move the body in any given range of flexibility is called mobility. Let's say you can flop down into the splits. You're very flexible, but that does not mean you have *mobility* throughout that whole range. If you had mobility in a full split, you would be able to stand on one foot and actively lift your other leg until you were standing in a full split. Ballerinas are the masters of mobility as they have the stability needed to control their bodies through vast ranges of flexibility. When flexibility training is done well, the stretching of muscles and fascia actually increases their elasticity, instead of putting force on the ligaments or joints.

WAYS TO INCREASE FLEXIBILITY

So many people go to the gym, or go for a run, or go for a hike, but far fewer will do even ten minutes of stretching before or afterwards. Yoga has brought increased awareness and new flexibility tools to people around the world, but these days even many yoga classes are built around intense poses that make you sweat and give you a workout, without building your flexibility.

Similar to strength, it helps to understand the mechanics that expand or limit your flexibility. Every person's body is wildly unique. Some people have tissues that allow for huge ranges of motions while others do not. Some people are born with very limber bodies and others are built with more inherent strength and have to work much harder to gain flexibility. All bodies respond differently to different types of practices based on the makeup of their muscles, bones, tissues, and the personality of the practitioner. Here are a few different approaches to flexibility that you can experiment with:

Active and Passive Flexibility Training

Passive flexibility is the act of releasing the body's tightness and tension while it is in a stretched position. Yin yoga, a slower, more gentle form of yoga, is a great example of this. This is a chill way to sit in one pose for a long time and let the flexibility come to you. Active flexibility, on the other hand, is the act of using your strength and muscular control to access and express your body's flexibility. The ballerina that lifts one leg into a full split while standing on the other is an example of active flexibility. There is not one way to gain flexibility. Active is not better than passive, just like push-ups are not better than pull-ups. Once you know your movement goals, you can choose what type of training and specific stretches will get you there.

Proprioceptive Neuromuscular Facilitation (PNF)

PNF is a technique utilized to improve muscular elasticity by blending active and passive stretching. In PNF there is a dance between isometric squeezing (resisting a stretch) for five to ten seconds, then surrendering into a deeper stretch. This can be done in yoga poses or in partner stretching.

Heat Treatment

Heat is one of the body's natural inflammatory responses and it can be very useful in helping your body open. There are many ways to generate heat, including physical activity, topical creams, massage pressure, saunas, baths, or being in a tropical environment. One of my best friends growing up was a very strong and stiff gymnast. Every practice, we would laugh at him as our coach literally sat on him, trying to get his body to open up. But then after practice, he would sit in a hot tub for fifteen minutes and be able to get into the splits. Every body is different to some degree, but all bodies obey the laws of physics and thermodynamics. Having a warm body will help in your journey to gaining flexibility.

TYPES OF FLEXIBILITY TRAINING IN ACROYOGA

Solo and Partner Yoga

Yoga has gained huge global acclaim for making people more flexible and improving their quality of life. *Hatha yoga* is a system that can help people increase flexibility, breath awareness, and life balance over time. This is a multidimensional approach to getting the most out of becoming more flexible. There are some limitations and drawbacks when doing traditional solo stretches. Actively using the muscles you are trying to stretch does not allow them to fully relax. On the other hand, partner stretching leverages your partner's body weight as a prop to help open your body while you can keep your own muscles relaxed and loose.

Massage

In massage the receiver can be 100 percent passive and allow another's strength to be applied to their soft, relaxed body. Even though there are huge benefits to this style of gaining flexibility, it is limited to the skill of the massage therapist and the awareness and honest feedback of the receiver.

AcroYoga for Base's Leg and Hip Flexibility

Tim Ferriss, a friend and student of the practice, shared this in his book *Tools of Titans,* about his flexibility gains: "[AcroYoga] helped my hips, knee issues, ankle flexibility, and athletically speaking [I've become] more mobile than when I was competing in wrestling." Tim's increases in flexibility came from doing AcroYoga, and

more specifically from doing L-base range of motion training. L-basing is a major innovation in gaining hip mobility because you get to use your partner's weight to help you increase your flexibility. Their weight warms your muscles and assists you in finding new mobility in a much shorter time than any of the other techniques listed above.

Therapeutic Flying for Flyer's Upper Body Flexibility

When a flyer is supported in the air, they gain access to new ways to release and stretch their body. There are many back bend variations, shoulder openers, spinal twists, and other ways you can increase flexibility and release tension in a flyer's upper body. In therapeutic flying we get to utilize gravity as our secret weapon, as gravity can put space back into the body and help restore balance between right and left as the body hangs. During flight, trust and maybe even laughter are exchanged to create the potential for emotional release that is tied to physical release.

HOW TO BUILD FLEXIBILITY

Define Your Goals

First off, you need to know what skills

you want to practice and where flexibility is needed to have ease and success in those particular movements. Depending on your goals, there are differences in warm-up, flexibility training, and recovery. They might all involve "stretching," but each has unique aims and techniques.

Get to Know Your Range of Motion

An important thing to note in flexibility training is that your body will tend to rely on the areas where it is already flexible. Imagine your spine like a bicycle chain. Over time, some parts of the chain develop rust, causing certain areas to stick and others to compensate by moving more. When you do a backbend, the lubricated parts of the chain bend with freedom, and the ones with rust do not. The more you understand where your body moves and where it does not, the better you can design your flexibility training around the rusty parts and make big gains over time. My advice is to take your time coming in and out of the poses, and *be patient*. Slow, steady progress is the way to create lasting change. One shoulder injury or hamstring tear can set you back many months, or worse, permanently limit some ranges of motion.

Stretch Daily

Consistency is the key to building flexibility. No three-hour yoga workshop will turn you into Gumby no matter how enlightened the teacher is. If you hope to experience more substantial gains, it's smarter to do fifteen minutes of yoga as part of your daily rhythm than one or two hard classes a week. Many people invest 480 minutes per day at work. As you learn to invest five to fifteen minutes per day in a few stretches, your life and flexibility will surely improve.

FLEXIBILITY TRAINING PITFALLS

If flexibility is not balanced with strength, instability in your joints can limit control at some points in your range of motion. This can lead to injuries to your joints, muscles, and connective tissue. From 2001–2014 there were an estimated 29,590 yoga-related injuries that warranted treatment in emergency rooms throughout the US. There *can* be too much of a good thing. One of the only things my Mexican grandma said in English was, "Hold your horses, Jay Jay." Don't force your body into flexibility; invite it and listen for the response to your invitation.

FLEXIBILITY TRAINING PRINCIPLES

1. Be Consistent.

You might be thinking, *Wait, this is a typo, I already read this.* No typo—and please read it again. It's the simple things that are often hardest to maintain.

Our bodies are consistently inconsistent. At times, we are limber and have freedom of movement. Other times, the body is tight and uncooperative. To help bring consistency to the body's volatility, we can implement daily routines, rituals, and habits that help us balance our flexibility with strength.

When you are ready for transformation, commit to a few postures that a good movement or yoga teacher suggests for you based on your flexibility and movement goals. Do them three times per week, three to six breaths per pose, minimum.

A three-to-twenty-minute daily practice can greatly change your body and mind, especially if you stick with it. Your body will thank you for the steady investments in flexibility and mobility, and in turn you will feel more gratitude for your body's new capabilities.

2. Practice All Roles.

As a base you might wonder, *Why is the flyer so scared?* As a flyer you might wonder, *Why is the base so shaky?* And as the spotter you might wonder, *Why are these two making everything so complicated!?*

As soon as you step into the other roles, you will understand what fear feels like, how hard it can be to balance another human, or how much calibration it takes for two people to move as one.

Being flexible and changing roles gives you firsthand visceral experience of what it is like for other people. It would be like a man cross-dressing and going to a bar to understand the kind of attention women receive in that environment.

Flexibility is not just for your hamstrings, it's for your world view as well. The more fixed we are in our identity the less we understand how others feel. Be willing to practice flexibility for the purpose of increasing compassion and refining behavior based on your direct experience.

3. Your Body Is Your Best Yoga Teacher.

Your yoga teacher does not have to live with any injuries you sustain caused by an error in their judgment, whereas you will learn from your every wise decision and every careless one. I have studied directly with some of the world's most respected yoga teachers, but as much as I trust their wisdom and years of experience, there is no teacher better for me than my body.

A *guru*—from *gu* (darkness) and *ru* (light)—is a person who is regarded as having great knowledge, wisdom, and authority in a certain area, and uses it to shine a light on the shadows of their student's practice.

I have experienced great depth in my practices because I surrendered deeply to my teachers. But at the same time, I always ran their ideas and philosophies through my personal laboratory and came back with questions if something did not align with what my body was telling me.

Trust yourself and know that any masterful teacher will not just instruct you, they will point you toward the path leading to your own insight. Our bodies are designed to give biofeedback, and it is our life's mission to learn how to listen to what is being communicated.

SOLO FLEXIBILITY PRACTICES

Active Flexibility Drill: Handstand (HS) Shoulder Flexibility Test

PROPS NEEDED:
WOODEN DOWEL, BROOMSTICK, OR HOCKEY STICK

This exercise will build your acrobatic potential as it will show you the relationship between your strength and flexibility, and between your shoulder mobility and rib mobility. It can serve as a tool to help you understand where you are strong and mobile and where you have work to do.

   Isolating actions like straightening the arms, opening the shoulders, and bringing the ribs down are all essential to many acrobatic skills. This *Handstand (HS) Shoulder Flexibility Test* is used by many coaches to identify areas of potential improvement in handstands.

FOUNDATION:
» Lie on your belly, arms stretched overhead, nose touching the floor.

BEGINNER:
» Hands **hold the dowel shoulder width** apart, arms as extended as possible but resting on the floor.

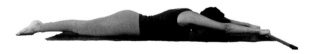

Arms Straight

INTERMEDIATE:

» Hands hold the dowel shoulder width apart, arms completely straight.
» **Lift your arms off the floor** toward the ceiling, reaching as high as possible with straight arms.

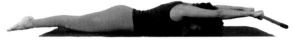

Hands off Floor

ADVANCED:

» Hands hold the dowel shoulder width apart, arms completely straight.
» Lift your arms off the floor toward the ceiling, **reaching as high as possible with straight arms**. The rest of the body stays tight, unified, and in a straight line with your nose touching the floor.
» *Hold for 10 seconds at the top of your range.*

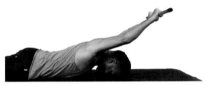

Hands Above Head

EXPERT:

» Lie on your back, hands hold the dowel shoulder width apart, arms completely straight.
» Bring your arms up and **have a partner press your lower ribs down** with clear and comfortable pressure.
» **With ribs in, bring backs of the hands toward the floor** slowly This teaches active flexibility with a boundary at the ribs so you learn to be hollow and find great shoulder alignment.

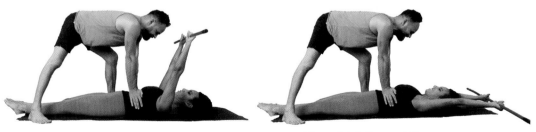

Partner Holds Ribs Down   Move Stick Toward Floor

Uttanasana (Ut): Standing Forward Fold

In AcroYoga, much of the practice happens with a base lying on the ground with their legs extended vertically. This is called L-basing and in this kind of acrobatics, the flyer's whole bodyweight is balanced on the base in various shapes and positions.

For many bases the key to easing into L-basing is to open their hamstrings. Often when people start with yoga or AcroYoga, their hamstrings can be very tight. This is why in Chapter 4, *Your First Flight*, using extra padding under the hips is recommended for bases who struggle with straightening their legs vertically.

This pose is diagnostic and helps you build the flexibility you need for success as a base.

BEGINNER:

» Stand up and fold over your legs, feet hip width apart, legs bent, **hands supported by yoga blocks**.

» *Hold for 3–5 breaths.*

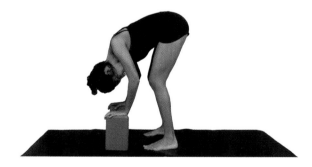

Forward Fold with Blocks

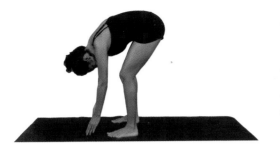

Legs Bent, Feet Apart

INTERMEDIATE:

» Stand up and fold over your legs, feet hip width apart, legs bent, **fingertips touching the floor.**

» *Hold for 3–5 breaths.*

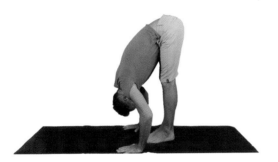

Legs Straight, Feet Together

ADVANCED:

» Stand up and fold over your legs, feet together, legs straight, **palms touching the floor.**

» *Hold for 3–5 breaths.*

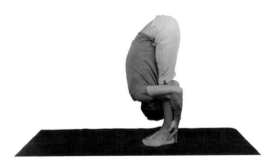

Full Forward Fold

EXPERT:

» Stand up and fold over your legs, feet together, legs straight, **hands holding your ankles** and face touching your shins.

» *Hold for 3–5 breaths.*

PARTNER FLEXIBILITY PRACTICE

Seated Partner Yoga Flow

Seated back to back partner stretches are a fun and easy way to open your body and invite communication and listening. When you tune into these qualities, your breaths will often become synchronized, soft, slow, and deep. This practice helps your focus stay in the present moment.

FOUNDATION:

> » Sit back to back with legs crossed.
> » Hands can touch the ground if needed to control the amount of weight in the stretches.

ACTIONS:

> » Lean sideways, backward, forward, and twist.
> » Breathe, communicate your needs, and listen to the feedback of your partner.
> » *Once warm, alternate pausing in each position for 3–5 breaths.*

VISIT **WWW.ACROYOGA.ORG/MCP** TO DOWNLOAD A FREE WORKBOOK, WATCH TUTORIALS, AND FIND OUR COMPANION VIDEO COURSE TO HELP YOU ACTIVATE THE PRINCIPLES AND PRACTICES DISCUSSED IN THIS CHAPTER.

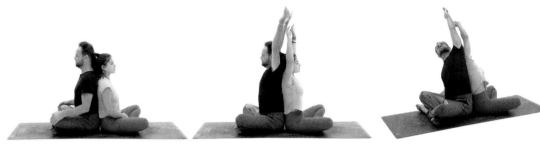

1. Sit Back to Back

2. Raise Arms Overhead

3. Side Bend: Reach
One Arm Up and Over

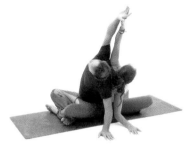

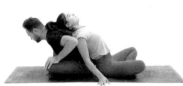

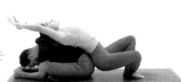

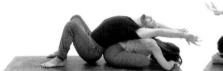

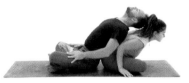

4. Side Bend:
Switch Direcitons

5. Forward & Back Bend

6. Forward & Back Bend:
Switch Directions

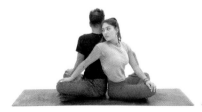

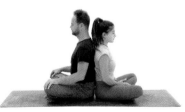

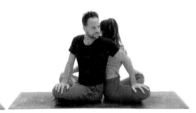

7. Arms Up & Offer More
Body Weight

8. Arms Up & Offer More
Body Weight: *Switch Directions*

9. Spinal Twist: Reach One
Arm to Partner's Knee

10. Spinal Twist:
Switch Directions

11. Meditation: Sit in Silence
and Breathe

REFLECT & EXPAND YOUR FLEXIBILITY

Flexibility Journaling is a practice that can unite the openness of the mind with the flexibility of the body. This prompt will help you sense the internal landscape of your soft spots and hard edges so that you can invite flexbility into your life where you need it most.

Outward Reflection

1. Write the name of someone you know who you think is very flexible.
2. What qualities does this "flexible" person have?

Inward Reflection

3. Where do I have flexibility and openness in my life?
4. Where in my life do I want more flexibility or openness?
5. What habit, practice, or quality would support flexibility in my relationships?

Make a Path Forward

6. What would success look like in my flexibility-building practice?
7. What skill or move would be a huge milestone for my expression of flexibility?
8. In pursuit of my goals, what exercises will I dedicate to, and for how long?

As an example, your strength journal might look something like this:

1. *Elyse.*
2. *She has ease in many movements, elegance, and a great ability to express...*
3. *I don't lock my house or car. My hips and shoulders are quite flexible.*
4. *I want to be more expressive in the ways I sing, dance, and dress. I would also like to open up my back more.*
5. *Being less controlling and more accepting of my friends' different ways of seeing/doing things would bring more flexibility into my relationships.*
6. *Success with my flexibility would look like being more consistent with my stretching and doing Wheel pose with less struggle.*
7. *A huge milestone for me would be doing a Back Walkover.*
8. *For the next month, I will stretch my back 3 times a week for 20 mins each, and do three Wheel poses at the end of each session. For my internal flexibility, I will express myself with dance or singing for 10 minutes a day. For my relationships I will practice more acceptance in conversation with my friends.*

PART III
YOUR MIND IS YOUR STRONGEST MUSCLE

At this stage in our journey together, you have had your first flight, seen the main building blocks of AcroYoga, and learned some ideas for building strength, increasing flexibility, and training smart. That's enough for years of growth, but we are about to go much further!

Now it's time to change your mind, find more balance, and become an acrobat. When most people see acrobatics, the default reaction is, *"That's amazing! I could never do that."* I have held people in the air as they did an acro skill, and still witnessed them yell with full conviction, *"I CAN'T DO THIS!"*

The mind is the first door to your practice that will lead you to many more doors and new possibilities in your life. Once an AcroYogi knows how to train their mind and balance their body, they have sown the two most important seeds for the growth of their acrobatics.

In this section you will take the Solar Elements of AcroYoga, mix them with the positivity of mental training, and add a bit of life philosophy. With this recipe you will be able to consistently blow your mind and your friends' minds with all the new things you will be able to do with them.

9

MENTAL TRAINING

Yoga is learning to stop how the mind turns things around.
—*YOGA SUTRAS OF PATAÑJALI*, 1.2, TRANSLATED BY GESHE MICHAEL ROACH

I met author and Tibetan Buddhist teacher Geshe Michael Roach in Hong Kong at the world's first Asia Yoga Conference in 2007. He was easy to spot because he had the biggest smile in the room. I had read his books *The Diamond Cutter* and *How Yoga Works* and was a huge fan of his work. I shyly went up to him and said, "I'm Jason and I loved reading your books." He responded, "Jason Nemer, the one that wrote the book on AcroYoga, I have your book too!" He continued, "I have very few possessions but this book is one of my greatest sources of happiness." I was blown away that he knew my work and was an AcroYogi. This man was the first Westerner to receive the esteemed title of Geshe, the Tibetan Buddhist honorific for "doctor." He is a deep practitioner and has done multiple three-year silent retreats where he studied ancient texts and brought them to life in his daily practices.

The way he has trained his mind and life, using Hindu and Buddhist philosophy, has influenced my own life and practices greatly. It was not one book, practice, or conversation we had that shifted me, but more so witnessing someone who has mastered their mind and seeing how they move through the world. Of course the laws of physics still govern his movement, but it's like he floats on a cloud above a lot of the shit most of us struggle with. He emits joy, peace, and skill in the way he approaches day-to-day life. Luckily for all of us, one of his greatest loves is sharing his passion for ancient philosophy and how to apply it practically. I have sprinkled his gems of wisdom throughout this book in an attempt to bring more context to the importance of the mind in unlocking and advancing your AcroYoga practice.

Many years of gymnastics training wired my brain in a particular way.

When I would get to the next skill in my journey, I had to face my fears and decide if I was ready to attempt the risk of a new skill. Once I decided I was ready, I would check in with my coach to see if they agreed. If they gave me the green light, I would ground my body and mind with one breath, giving 100 percent of my trust to my body. Then I would attempt the skill with full belief that I could do it. I was right more times than I was wrong, due to amazing coaching and a clear mental state. This was my recipe for reaching my goal of going to the Olympics. I knew early on that no goal was too big, and each day I rallied my body and mind into a place of union around that reality.

As humans and AcroYogis, our potential is infinite. In this chapter I'll share my perspective and the views of various wisdom traditions on understanding the mind and harnessing mental adaptability to open yourself to greater possibility.

OUR COMMAND CENTER

The human brain weighs around three pounds, or less than 2 percent of our total bodyweight. It is the central command center for our entire body. With all this power it is also responsible for shaping our potential for suffering or happiness. The view that our thoughts can create suffering or happiness is a primary principle of the *Yoga Sūtras of Patañjali*. A known disciple of yoga in the West and a well-studied guru, Sri Swami Satchidananda said the following about the mind in the context of the *Yoga Sūtras:*

> There are, of course, many western approaches to the study and control of the mind, each advancing various different concepts and techniques. But compared to these, the ancient Yogic science has more data points due to the element of time. For thousands of years the yogis have probed the mysteries of the mind and consciousness, and we may well discover that some of their findings are applicable to our own search as well.

Both ancient yogis like Patañjali and modern neuroscientists know that we actively participate in shaping how our brain is wired. When you change your brain, you change your life. Your mental activity is constantly creating new neural pathways based on your thoughts. Yogis say, "Where attention goes, energy flows." When we intentionally direct the flow of energy and information through these neural circuits, we not only directly alter the brain's activity, we actually alter its physical structure, too. You can think of your thoughts like push-ups that grow the muscles of the brain. The more awareness you have of your thoughts, the more you affect how your brain functions, thereby dictating how you experience and interact with the world.

Is there a right way to see the world? What are the traps that keep your mind stuck? How can you stop turning things around in your mind? You can use AcroYoga as a tool to explore these questions, sharpen your focus, and change your worldview with new neural pathways.

CONDITIONS OF THE MIND

Mental Strength

Yes we can.
—PRESIDENT BARACK OBAMA

Every day we can choose what we think, say, and do with greater clarity.

A strong mind does not look for limits or the reasons why something will not work. A strong mind sees a possibility and believes in the ability to reach that vision. When we align with the power of the mind, we greatly increase our chances of getting what we want out of life. In AcroYoga, I've seen countless people reframe negative and limiting beliefs such as "I can't do that," into "I can't do that, yet." Even further evolved is, "I can do that if I get stronger," or, "We can do that if we get a good spotter." The body will follow the anthem of the mind.

Mental Flexibility

If the brain is the cause of suffering he can also be its cure.
—DALAI LAMA

Mental flexibility means being able to see things from different perspectives and, when appropriate, adjust your thoughts, beliefs, and the way you relate. Change is a universal constant that should encourage pivots in how we think. The ability to change your mind once you learn new information is a superpower. When we lack mental flexibility we are unable to alter our conclusions even after receiving new evidence or input.

We can choose to see the world as something that we navigate and deal with as individuals, or we can open ourselves to the possibility that our world is created in collaboration with the people around us. One of the best ways to explore this concept through AcroYoga is to attempt a skill in your non-dominant role. If you usually base, try doing the skill as a flyer, and vice versa. Putting yourself in another person's shoes will drive home the way in which you are each co-creating the other person's experience, and can give you a whole new level of compassion and insight into your partner's point of view.

The ability to change your mind is one of the skills you will learn practicing AcroYoga. When we are part of a community of people practicing the same skills, we feel more supported in actualizing our dreams.

Mental Struggle

The mind flies off, and with that comes pain in the body, unhappy thoughts, shaking in the hands, and other parts of the body; the breath falling in and out of rhythm as it passes in and out.

—*YOGA SUTRAS OF PATAÑJALI*, 1.31
TRANSLATED BY GESHE MICHAEL ROACH

The emotional state captured in the quote above is something I am confident most of us have experienced by the time we reach adulthood. These are symptoms that occur when there are disturbances in the mind. Because everyone has a different recipe for what makes them happy, there is no one way to define happiness. In life there will be moments when we are blissfully happy and others when we are explosively upset. So much of our suffering is theoretical, and involves things that may or may not even happen.

When it's time for my dental checkup and I am sitting in the dentist's chair, I always treat it as a master yoga class. The dentist is there drilling and drilling. Left unchecked, my mind will freak out: "Oh shit! He will hit a nerve soon and it will hurt so bad." When I get my monkey mind under control, I know how blessed I am to have a highly trained human with high-tech gadgets working to prevent future pain and suffering. Knowing that, going through a bit of discomfort right now becomes more tolerable. I can hate going to the dentist and fear what might happen, or I can be grounded in the reality that modern dentistry is generally safe, effective, and a privilege. Whichever way I think about it determines my very different levels of suffering or happiness. This is all in my control if I practice with awareness.

Mental Focus

Practice of fixing the mind on one object should be performed to eliminate these disturbances.
—*YOGA SUTRAS OF PATAÑJALI,* 1.32
TRANSLATED BY GESHE MICHAEL ROACH

It is healthy to give our minds a "timeout" when we want to change and heal. In those moments, sit down, stop doing so much, and give your mind and body time to connect with each other. AcroYoga poses can serve as medicine for an unbalanced or scattered mental state. When you are balancing a human or being balanced by another human, there are not many other places your mind can be other than right there in your body and in full presence and connection with the other. The confines of a still body collaborating with another can allow the weaker parts of our minds to quiet, allowing the clearer, stronger messages to come through. In Chapter 15, *Everything Can Be a Meditation*, I provide many more ideas and practices on how to

use meditation as a tool to heal and strengthen your mind.

YOUR MIND EXPANDS OR CONTRACTS YOUR POTENTIAL

Countless seeds within our minds make us see the great variety of things around us.
—*YOGA SUTRAS OF PATAÑJALI,* 4.24
TRANSLATED BY GESHE MICHAEL ROACH

A seed can live a long time in its shell. It takes the right conditions to sprout. In that tender stage the roots move past many obstacles to find a stable place to take hold. Then the leaves search for nourishment via sunlight. Words are like seeds that we plant in our minds. Words are our minds' best attempt to describe and understand the vastly chaotic world around us. A key strength in words is that they can be passed on between generations, and ideas can then germinate around the world.

Your native language is one of the determining factors in which seeds you have available to plant in the garden of your mind. This is the worldview from your ancestors that has been passed down to you. Many words and concepts exist in all languages: hungry, hot, cold, food, water, like, dislike, sun, moon, angry, funny, etc. There are also many words and concepts that are unique to certain languages. The Hawaiian language has many words for lava. The Inuit have many words for snow. Their physical environment has dictated a need for words and concepts that other cultures do not need.

Our thoughts drastically affect our language, and in turn our language affects how we think. Another example of this is a story about the Dalai Lama: He was working with some Westerners and they were describing the feeling of self-hate. He even asked for a few different interpreters to try to explain this concept to him. It was a concept he had never heard of, and for him there was no basis for this state of being. Know that while there are intrinsic human ideas that we all share, many concepts are not universal. Communication and listening are the keys to expanding our understanding of different people and different ideas.

AcroYoga brings the mind into the present moment to transform our understanding of what we are capable of in partnership. We push our mental horizons as we do yoga on the edge with one another. Your AcroYoga partnerships can support the growth of your mental

seeds from ideas to real things in your life. As much as we are spotters for the safety and well-being of the physical body, we can also spot one another's words and actions. If a partner says, "I always fall from my handstands, I suck at them," I might encourage them by saying, "You've gotten much better at handstands in the last few months! I am happy to help you balance, but if you think you suck I won't be able to help you as much until you change that story."

A good coach will ask the right questions and reflect the ideas needed to invite the student to change their mind and plant the right mental seeds. Once a thought has taken root, it can become a strong anchor in your mind, be it positive or negative. One mango seed can, with the right conditions, rain down thousands of mangos. This is why it is key to be aware of which seeds you plant—which words you use—so you can crack the right ones open and let them take root in your life.

We must become gardeners.
—*YOGA SUTRAS OF PATAÑJALI*, 4.3
TRANSLATED BY GESHE MICHAEL ROACH

Usually gardeners grow the foods and plants that they enjoy eating. Regardless of what they grow, every garden needs weed control and sometimes unwanted things grow in unwanted places. The mind can be a very fruitful garden if it's well maintained, or it can become a wild forest of pesky weeds and things you don't want to harvest. You love mangos— the tropical juiciness moves your soul, but hate Brussels sprouts—you are still recovering from childhood traumas of being forced to eat these dwarfed cabbages. When you think or speak about mangos, you are germinating a plant you love in your mind. Sometimes we exhibit a strong pattern of negative thoughts. "I am not good enough for my partner," is one, for example. Once you manifest that thought, a negativity plant (Brussels sprouts) begins growing and taking up space in your mind. This reduces how much space the other positive plants (mangos) can occupy in your mind.

If you can trace back to when and where you first planted that seed, you have the potential to cut it out of your fertile mind. Surprisingly, the opposite is also true. When did I start believing that I am beautiful and sexy? It was when my girlfriend affirmed clearly how much she was attracted to me, and that relationship allowed me to plant and grow a big ass mango tree of self-confidence. Surround yourself with other farmers that you love and trust and start cultivating the beautiful garden of your dreams.

The storehouse is planted by the things we do.
—*YOGA SUTRAS OF PATAÑJALI*, 2.12
TRANSLATED BY GESHE MICHAEL ROACH

From the seeds of our thoughts come words, and from words we eventually harvest the fruit in our actions. When these three expressions of reality are in harmony, we are doing yoga. We are in a state of union with ourselves. Nobody but you can know if your thoughts, words, and actions are in harmony. It takes sensitivity with your mental states and dedication to the actions that follow to reach this kind of yogic harmony. Achieving this state within allows you to listen deeply to yourself, and with more discernment, to the world around you.

HOW WE LISTEN

Your actions speak so loudly, I cannot hear what you are saying.
—RALPH WALDO EMERSON

The brain receives millions of electrochemical signals from our sensory organs and does its best to interpret them. One of the main functions of the brain is to classify the world around it. That is done by observation and compartmentalization. Cultivating deep listening is one of the most powerful learning aids I have encountered. There is a reason we were given two ears and one mouth. Listening is not just a practice for the ears, it's a full-body sport! With practice all of our senses can be taught to listen, providing us with incredibly valuable information about our surroundings.

Talking without listening is not communication—it's noise. Communication entails so much more. Couples or friends who have known each other for years can hold full conversations through subtle gestures or facial expressions. Tears, laughter, and sighs can all transmit more powerful messages than words ever could. In massage the reflexive responses of the body clearly communicate when tension is being released or when pressure is too strong. Expanding our listening capacity to encompass all the senses is key to becoming a perceptive human and a successful AcroYogi.

There are many tools available to anyone wishing to become more receptive.

Our ability to listen is greatly affected by how interested we are in the subject; once you are aware of what excites you, the rest of the journey is learning tools and then applying them. When we strengthen our listening skills, we support others to express a much wider spectrum of their human experience. This rich spectrum ranges from describing the taste of a mango to expressing grief and heartbreak or unconditional love. Deep listening and clear communication support the sharing of information, and with that exchange often comes understanding.

Understanding is always a work in progress that should be subject to change and revision. We often misunderstand due to not knowing what another is really thinking. In our modern lives we have, to a large degree, left behind many senses that used to be more central in our approach to relating with each other. Intuition, mysticism, and magic are also parts of our being that can help us relate to more esoteric aspects of human life. Simply because you cannot describe everything with words or measure it with scientific instruments does not mean it does not exist. Just because you cannot understand something fully with your mind does not mean it does not have value. To reach deeper levels of understanding, we must become good listeners.

HOW WE SEE

Knowing you don't know is wholeness. Thinking you know is a disease. Only by recognizing that you have an illness can you move to seek a cure. The Master is whole because she sees her illnesses and treats them, and thus is able to remain whole.

—LAO TZU, *TAO TE CHING*, CHAPTER 71

What Lao Tzu is trying to highlight in this quote is that the fullness or emptiness of our knowledge cup deeply affects our life. The more perspectives from which we can look at something, the more open we are to seeing things as they really are. The mental lens or system we use to process information shapes our worldview and gives order to chaos. There are many systems, some ancient and some more recent, that can help us understand how to navigate the complexities of life. I see these systems like prescription glasses; each lens allows you to see things a little differently and hopefully more clearly. Some of them

include Western medicine, Traditional Chinese Medicine (TCM), Fox News, Taoism, Catholicism, communism, the Spanish language, *Hatha* Yoga, modern science, etc. These systems can color your perception of reality. Understanding this and knowing which lenses to use in various situations can support your harmonious and efficient progress toward your training and life goals. Empty your cup, try on a beginner's mind, and let your practice and your community teach you about becoming the best you can be.

Risk and Worry

Worrying is praying for what you don't want.
—BHAGAVAN DAS

Risk is part of being alive and it can bring us closer to death. Risk is exciting and sexy and sometimes scary. Worry is about the future and if you are reading this, you are probably fine on most levels. You are alive, and worrying about whatever you are worrying about does not change the situation at hand. This isn't to suggest that all worrying is valueless. Some worry can lead to logical troubleshooting which can be smart and soothing to the mind. But most worrying does not. The more you worry about something the more invasive seeds you are planting in your mental garden. Find the root cause of why you are worrying. What is provoking this flood of bad seeds you don't want or need in your garden?

The more you learn about your true potential as a human and the more you practice and build your skills, the better you will become at assessing risk. As you improve at assessing risk you'll find yourself able to take on bigger risks with less worry because your abilities and confidence support those decisions. Two questions to always ask yourself are: "What will I lose if I don't worry?" and "What will I gain if I let go of worry?"

HOW WE LEARN

I hear and I forget, I see and I remember, I do and I understand.
—CONFUCIUS

Learning and Practicing

Our minds are built to learn. Learning is like putting a bit of food in our mouths. Practice is chewing up that bite, and integration is digesting it. If we only learn without practicing, we will have a mouth full of food that we cannot hope to swallow. If we only practice a few things, we might need new morsels to whet our appetite and help us develop a hunger for new flavors.

In-formation

An essential nutrient for our brains, other than oxygen and glucose, is information. We constantly receive signals from our sensory organs taking in the outside world as our brains interpret the information. Any conclusions we have about life and the world are not fixed, they are ideas that are *in formation*. Our ancestors tried to point to this by calling our key brain food "in-formation." It is ever growing, changing, and flowing, like us.

Knowledge and Wisdom

Children learn rapidly because everything is new and full of wonder to them. The more knowledge we accumulate, the more likely we are to become rigid in our thoughts and less open to the mysteries of life. There is the learning of concrete things and names, and there is also the learning that happens on a deeper level when the mind quiets down and becomes witness to the magic of the world. Knowledge is merely theoretical. It becomes wisdom when our wonder leads us to test it in the real world.

Instruction and Education

There are two main ways people teach: instruction and education. Instruction is putting a structure inside a student's mind. Mental structures are frameworks to help us understand and predict the chaos of the world. The next step, education, is what we can evolve toward. The root of the word "educate" is *educere*, which means "to bring out." In instruction we put in information, and with education we bring out what is inherent. For example, if I instruct you in how to spot five different skills and you drill them for months with flawless execution, you can then tap into your own wellspring of wisdom that reaches far beyond those five initial skills. From this level of embodied experience you can know how to spot a new skill by leaning into your educated guesses.

EMPTINESS AND PROJECTION

Stay in that one pure thought, and never forget it; that single most important thing: things are empty of being what they are by themselves.

—*YOGA SUTRAS OF PATAÑJALI*, 1.43
TRANSLATED BY GESHE MICHAEL ROACH

There are many ways to perceive the world. One option is to think of the world like a movie we are watching, with each day unfolding scene by scene on a blank screen. Another more Buddhist perspective is that rather than simply watching the movie, we are making it, or projecting it ourselves onto the blank screen. To see the truth in this perspective, take this example: Imagine you are watching your favorite basketball team in their final game with five seconds to go. You and your best friend are fans of opposing teams. In the final seconds, your favorite player sinks a three-pointer to win it all! You are ecstatic, celebrating the best moment of the year. In the same moment, your friend drops to his knees in despair. The game-winning shot was not good or bad; it was neutral, empty. But you projected meaning onto it based on your life, your experiences, your preferences and aversions. In this sense, the mind shapes our experience of reality.

If you're training handstands and exit your handstand attempt earlier than expected, your spotter might ask why you gave up on your handstand. What they don't know is that your wrist was in pain so you came down to avoid further aggravating it. Without realizing it, your spotter may incorrectly paint in the details of why you exited early. While we may not write the script or direct the other actors, our worldview powerfully determines whether the "movie of our lives" is a comedy, tragedy, horror, or an epic drama.

NOBLE ELEMENTS OF THE MIND

These Noble Elements are specific to the mental states found through a harmonious and joyful AcroYoga practice. They can also be cultivated in relationships in your everyday life. When you practice with full intention, the following elements will be present.

Communication (Co)

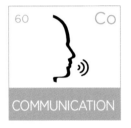

Communication is a practice that ranges from being suppressed to expressed to the outside world. It implies the sharing of energy and ideas that can be conveyed in many different ways. Our bodies express through movement and touch. Spirit is expressed through song, dance, and ritual. Our minds express through words—both written and spoken. Beyond words, communication between people can happens with sounds, gestures, facial expressions, and eye contact.

Expression is key to letting the world know our precious gifts and who we truly are. In AcroYoga, we work on being clear with communication in acrobatics and honest with our needs in therapeutics.

Listening (Li)

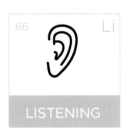

Listening is the silent skill that does most of the heavy lifting in relationships. The spectrum of listening ranges from being closed off to fully open. We are social animals that, by design, love to connect with others on many levels.

There are as many ways to build relationships as there are people on earth, but listening will be a steady pillar in the building and nurturing of any of your relationships.

Both communication and listening are acquired skills that take time to fully bloom, and always have room to grow. The willingness to listen must be present for us to learn things, and this is important because we are naturally invested in learning—it is one of the most satisfying treats for our monkey mind.

Understanding (Un)

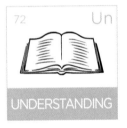

Understanding is the fruit of communication paired with listening. When we understand, we feel safe. When we feel safe, we can power down our fight-or-flight centers, allowing us access to more creative, joyful states of being. Understanding is another word for love. Without understanding, there can be no compassion. It is the baseline for all relationships.

Understanding is predominately a mental concept. That being said, the mind can also understand emotions and abstract spiritual ideas. In Thai, the word "understand" translates literally to "enters my heart." In English, when you know something well you say you know it by heart.

These clues help us see that understanding lives in different levels of our being. Curiosity paves the path to understanding; when we follow curiosity to knowledge, our capacity to understand finds its conclusion.

Do I not destroy my enemies when
I make them my friends?

—ABRAHAM LINCOLN

MENTAL TRAINING PRINCIPLES

1. Know Thyself.

Knowing who you are is a moving target because each day life teaches you something new about yourself. The practice of yoga is designed to mine the gems of your soul and help you find ways to activate them in your life.

Imagine someone with very little self-knowledge. I see them as a human with sharp edges and little bits of explosives hidden in the cracks. When someone does or says something that they don't agree with, they blow up. Yoga can smooth out your rough edges by teaching you to keep your cool in challenging poses. This capacity then translates to other situations in your life.

The deeper your self-knowledge, the easier it can be to align and heal all the parts of you. Those parts include your joints, muscles, and organs. They also include your pain, your worldview, your emotions, fears, and dreams. To become whole, you must dedicate yourself to self-study and continue doing the daily work to become better friends with yourself.

2. Align Your Mind.

Thinking, speaking, and moving are all very different forms of interacting with the world, but they are all driven from the same command center. Our mind is the holder of our ideas, words, and dance steps.

Due to the vast nature of what we contain as humans, it's easy to get lost in any one aspect of who we are or what we do. We all know someone who is super introverted and can spend hours "in their head." Or we have a friend who talks without thinking. Or maybe worse: a friend who acts without thinking.

Yogis dedicate themselves to aligning the three dimensions of thoughts, words, and actions in order to attain harmony and balance with themselves and the outside world.

3. The Mind Changes First.

It takes seven to ten years for the cells in our bodies to regenerate, with the exception of our brain cells: In adult brains, most neurons change their connections with other neurons rather than regrowing, and the electrochemical impulses that signal between them take approximately one millisecond to travel.

With speeds like that, in a full day of new thoughts and ideas we can have drastic shifts in our brains and our lives. Even though our bodies take years to physically change, our minds do not; what we believe can change in a millisecond.

As much as life can be predictable, it is also built on dichotomies, extremes, and paradoxes. We can use this to our advantage by shifting how we see the world and how quickly and often we allow ourselves to evolve our beliefs.

MENTAL TRAINING PRACTICES

These practices are designed to bring awareness to and shift your mental habits. Carve out a little bit of time to spend with each practice and keep them in your back pocket. The more frequently you incorporate these, the easier it will become for you to change your mind, say what you mean, and let your actions spring forth from a place of alignment with your thoughts and words.

Change Your Thoughts

Becoming aware of negative thought patterns and limiting beliefs can help you redirect your mental energy. To get familiar with choosing different thoughts that uplift you instead of limit you, try this journaling exercise:

Pick three beliefs you want to change, and for each negative thought, find its antidote.

For example:
- » *"I'm too big to fly,"* changes to, *"I will find strong bases."*
- » *"I suck at handstands,"* changes to, *"I am dedicated to improving my handstand."*
- » *"I have a bad back,"* changes to, *"My back is inviting more mindfulness and care."*

In the *Yoga Sūtras*, these are examples of what Patañjali calls *praktipaksha bhavana*, which means "to cultivate counteracting thoughts." When negative thoughts in the mind are swirling, you can choose to focus on something different. With practice and time, the mind will start to operate in a more peaceful state.

Say What You Mean

Be intentional with the words you choose to better guide how you feel and how you interact with others. Journal about any "always" and "never" statements that you tend to make, things you think you can't do, and negative statements you want to shift.

> » "Always" and "never" statements are hardly ever true! (*"You always drop me!" "You never catch me!"* etc.)
> » Reorient from saying "I can't" to "I can't—yet."
> » Change negative associations like *"my bad knee"* or *"my bad side"* to lighthearted ones like *"my magic knee, my fun side, my second favorite side."*

Take Daily Action

When you move into action, you involve your whole being as part of the seed of thought taking root and flowering. Find three things per day you will do to support you in moving toward your goals.

For example:
> » *I will journal about flexibility to help me change the way I think and speak about it.*
> » *I will take a hot shower or bath to open my body.*
> » *After the bath I will stretch for ten minutes.*

VISIT *WWW.ACROYOGA.ORG/MCP* TO DOWNLOAD A FREE WORKBOOK, WATCH TUTORIALS, AND FIND OUR COMPANION VIDEO COURSE TO HELP YOU ACTIVATE THE PRINCIPLES AND PRACTICES DISCUSSED IN THIS CHAPTER.

10

BALANCE ☯

As it acts in the world, the Tao is like the bending of a bow. The top is bent downward, the bottom is bent up. It adjusts excess and deficiency so that there is perfect balance. It takes from what is too much and gives to what isn't enough. Those who try to control, who use force to protect their power, go against the direction of the Tao. They take from those who don't have enough and give to those who have far too much. The Master can keep giving because there is no end to her wealth. She acts without expectation, succeeds without taking credit, and doesn't think she is better than anyone else.
—LAO TZU, *TAO TE CHING*, CHAPTER 77

Lao Tzu was the founder of Taoism and his book, the *Tao Te Ching*, contains eighty-one short chapters that can be read in a day. I have been reading this little book over and over for almost twenty years, and every time I pick it up I find more meaning and depth. Fundamental to Taoism is balance, represented by the yin-yang symbol, seen here in the chapter title. In his chapter on balance, Lao Tzu writes about dualism—good and bad, high and low, right and wrong, love and hate—and how the full complexity of the world does not fit into these boxes because they leave no room for the vast nuances of nature.

One way to understand balance is by recognizing that within all things are opposing poles, and by expanding your awareness of the extremes, you can find your happy place between them. Let's say we are talking about massage pressure. Maybe you have only had very middle-of-the-road massages. (I call them "spa massages.") They want you to feel good, but they are not really invested in digging deeper into places of stored trauma. On the opposing poles of soft massage and strong massage, we can compare a Reiki healer to a deep tissue therapist. Reiki practitioners do not actually touch you, whereas a deep tissue massage therapist might push you to the point of screaming. Once you have experienced the range of both extremes, you have a greater capacity to find your sweet spot with massage and to be more comfortable across a broader range of experiences as your understanding of pressure expands.

Still, once you find your sweet spot between the extremes, that is always subject to change, as all things are in our natural world. In university my Asian Philosophy teacher said, "All things change. Can anyone give me an example of something that does not change?" I was eager to make an impression and threw up my hand with enthusiasm: "My love for my mother has not changed. I loved her when I was born, as a child, and still today I love her." I was so proud of myself for stumping the teacher, or so I thought. He replied, "So as a baby you loved suckling her breast, as a child you loved her for giving you toys, and today you love her for paying your tuition. Your love for your mother has and will always change." I was captivated by the philosophical smackdown that was delivered by this man and the roots of his wisdom, which emanated from the yin-yang symbol.

I kept the teaching of this symbol with me as I deepened my healing practices.

The more I learned about the body through yoga and doing therapeutic treatments, the more I began to realize how imbalanced the human body is by design. The heart is on our left side; most of us are right- or left-handed; there is a football-sized liver in the upper right side of our abdomen, a spleen on the left, etc. Then we go out and live our lives, throwing all kinds of new chaos at our bodies in the hope and expectation that it will handle everything and continue to work for us every day. Finding equilibrium is essential to mitigating the stressors we are exposed to on all the levels. Balance increases lifespan and quality of life. It is the fountain of youth.

Many of us will live the first half of our lives in reasonably good health regardless of how well we take care of ourselves. But in the second half of our lives we will be supported or challenged by the habits and routines we built in the first half. Good habits accumulated over years create more ease as we age; bad habits accumulated over years create more dis-ease as we age. When people die prematurely, it is often the result of a weakness in one of their organs due to strong imbalances. When people live life with balance their systems are more likely to function harmoniously, with no big health crises or need for interventions.

In its essence, balance is the practice of finding and refining your center, knowing that your center is not a static place. Balance is a dynamic state and when it is found the resulting sense of ease and calm is unmistakable. It's hard to find and easy to lose, but the magic of balance is in the presence you cultivate as you are searching for it. This chapter will give you some tools for bringing balance to your body and your lifestyle. Enjoy the ride!

PHYSICAL BALANCE

Physical balance can be regarded in terms of your food intake, amount and types of daily movement, quality of sleep, and organ function; then there is the actual practice of balancing, like walking on a tightrope. Your sight, inner ear, and ability to listen to where you stack your weight over points of support are all ingredients in physically balancing your body or your partner.

Seeing is believing: whether in a handstand or balancing your friend over your head, to find ease in physical balance, use your eyes when you can. To see for yourself how useful your sight is, try balancing on one foot, then close your eyes!

The inner ear contains highly sensitive organs for equilibrium. Its three semicircular canals are arranged at right angles to each other, so that they can sense motion in all three planes. In the canals are hair-like cells that respond to the flow of the endolymph fluid caused by movement of the head in any direction. They transmit signals indicating changes of position through the vestibular nerve.

Most people do the majority of their balance practices on their feet; walking, climbing stairs, running, jumping, and landing all begin and end with, to some degree, balancing your full body weight on your feet. What you learn on your feet is more or less the same on your hands, so listen closely to what your feet do to understand how to balance better on your hands.

Right in the Middle

There are many applications of the concept of "right in the middle." On a physical level, balancing on your feet or hands is done with maximum ease and efficiency when you are pouring your weight through the middle of your foundation. If your weight is forward in your fingers or toes, you have to grip with your muscles; if your weight is mostly in the heel of your palm or foot, you are on the verge of falling off the cliff with no parachute.

Wherever you are on the spectrum between strength and flexibility, your movement practices will benefit by you moving toward a fifty-fifty balance. If you have more strength than flexibility, shift your training to give those big muscles more potential to be expressed. If you are more flexible than strong, go to a CrossFit class and build some fire to fuel your amazing potential. So many times in life and in your practices, you are "right" when you are in the middle.

Sitting and Hanging

Sitting is a part of modern life for all of us—from our commute, to our desks at work, to eating; even going to the bathroom forces us to sit! When we sit we encourage non-optimal patterns in our hips, lower back, and neck. The World Health Organization has already identified physical inactivity as "the fourth biggest killer on the planet—sitting too much." It has been linked to a range of health issues including increased risk of heart attack, obesity, high blood pressure, high blood sugar, excess body fat, abnormal cholesterol levels, and cancer. Our biology dictates that if you don't use it, you lose it. Everything in the human body works on feedback.

In contrast to sitting, the action of hanging takes advantage of gravity to stretch and decompress our ape-like arms and shoulders. Simply by hanging we can create a template for better posture, open our shoulders and entire spinal column, and allow the front of our hips to open, which is important because chronic sitting shortens our hip flexors. The grip strength and wrist traction in hanging also helps to combat our texting thumbs and typing fingers. If you sit most of the day, try incorporating hanging into your routine and see if you notice a difference in your own body.

Pushing and Pulling

As acrobats and yogis we are pushers: the vast majority of the physical activities we do involve extending our arms and then pushing through them. In pushing practices the joints get compressed; in pulling they get tractioned. Knowing this can help you maintain balance in your upper body.

As you get hooked on AcroYoga, go to a park with some bars, get a doorway pull-up bar, or go to a gym that has a bar and get your pulling on! The simple act of pulling reduces our overall risk of injury because it balances our pushing strength, and as you just learned, the traction of hanging is therapy for the body.

Standing and Inverting

We are built to walk long distances. Standing in one place was not part of our Stone Age movement patterns. If you find yourself in a job or situation where you are standing for many hours, it can be helpful to balance one extreme with another. When you stand, your heart has to pump blood uphill to your thirsty brain, while your biggest muscles (in your legs and butt) use lots of blood that must be pumped uphill once again.

On the opposing pole from standing is inverting. Headstand (hs), Forearm Stand (4A), and Handstand (HS) are great ways for people who stand too much to find balance. As soon as you invert, meaning you get your head below your heart, it's all downhill, smooth sailing, and your heart goes on a mini vacation.

Physiologically speaking, standing and inverting are two extreme states of being that are very well suited for each other. Inverting balances the blood flow and instantly takes the weight of prolonged standing off the feet and lower back. The organs in our midsection—liver, spleen, kidneys, stomach, heart, and lungs—all hang in a new way, stretching the tissues and stimulating the movement of blood and other vital fluids.

Our perspective is literally turned on its head, so for those few precious breaths we see the world from a new vantage point. This vantage point demands a level of presence that standing upright does not. Because we are in a less familiar plane of existence, we are more sensitive and able to receive the benefits of slowing down and doing less. We all have movement patterns that are affected by our work, our past injuries, and our daily habits. When we go upside down in an inversion or therapeutic flight, we can experience magical moments where gravity helps bring our body back into optimal alignment.

LIFESTYLE BALANCE

Balance activity with serenity, wealth with simplicity, persistence with innovation, community with solitude, familiarity with adventure, constancy with change, leading with following.
—JONATHAN LOCKWOOD HUIE

There are entire sections of bookstores and online marketplaces dedicated to helping people balance their physical body's health. Here I will offer you ideas and philosophies you can apply to maximize the inner harmony of your life.

Work, Play, and Sleep

I like the eight-hour rule as a baseline: Start by designating eight hours each for work, play, and sleep each day. It's simple and not simple, which is the signature feeling of balance practices—easy to stick to for a day or two, but difficult to follow through with in the long term.

You may find that eight isn't the exact number for you, so adjust accordingly. For example, I do very well on seven hours of sleep, so maybe I will get to play for nine?! Also, defining what counts as work and play is an important and potentially difficult part of this task. I fly humans for a living—is that work or play? What about the "boring" tasks of life—cooking, cleaning, laundry—where are those hours logged? Can you turn those activities into games? Can you authentically enjoy doing the mundane things in life?

Even asking yourself these questions and looking at how much time you spend doing things each day is a worthwhile investment of your attention. Where AcroYoga can help is by bringing more play into your daily life. Not many adults get enough time playing. As a society we are very serious, and it is a beautiful practice to set time aside to have fun.

Active and Passive

If we are always on the go, the moments when we allow ourselves to fully relax can be life-changing. If we are more on the slothy end of the spectrum, movement and action can be similarly fulfilling. We can learn from contrast. Functionally, this is usually a question of finding the right balance between our movement practices and recovery, but it could also mean thinking about what our day-to-day lives require of us and finding ways to complement that with other types of activities.

For example, if you work at the farmers' market or as a nurse in a hospital, you are on your feet all day. Doing inversions with your friends after work or lying on your back with your feet up on the wall as you listen to some chill music could be your medicine. Alternatively, if you sit for eight hours at work, your body is craving any and all movements that look nothing like being in a chair. So don't go to the gym to sit on a bench as you lift weights. At the least if you do, add something else that contrasts your many hours of daily sitting. AcroYoga offers a great variety of shapes and movements that can break you out of the trap of sedentary life.

BALANCE TRAINING PITFALLS

It is possible when people get attached to a balanced, zen-like lifestyle that the inevitability of life throwing curveballs can pull them out of their happy place. It is all well and good to love drinking a perfectly steeped cup of organic tea from a handmade clay pot. But every once in a while, life might oblige you to accept an instant coffee in a Styrofoam cup. Being attached to any ideal, including balance, is not what *real balance* is about. Rather than attempting to control life in order to maintain the illusion of perfect balance, we need to learn to roll with the punches without getting knocked off our feet.

Water is fluid, soft, and yielding. But water will wear away rock, which is rigid and cannot yield. As a rule, whatever is fluid, soft, and yielding will overcome whatever is rigid and hard. This is another paradox: what is soft is strong.

—LAO TZU

BALANCE PRINCIPLES

1. Lose It to Find It.

Balance is a dynamic, living, moving thing. When we are physically balancing our own bodies or the bodies of our partners, we ebb and flow from being perfectly aligned, stable, and right in the sweet spot, to drifting away from this miraculous point. As we fall in and out of balance we get biofeedback that lets us know how much force we need to maintain the pose.

If we think we are perfectly aligned and do not explore the micro adjustments available from that point, we might be in a false sweet spot. Life is about trying to get to the best spot we can while having the courage to explore outside of that zone to see if things can get even better. If we cling to a purely middle path in life, we are not really living as fully as we can.

While there is nothing wrong with testing out the extremes of life, it is also not recommended or sustainable to live in those extremes. Being in balance is defined by knowing where the extremes are and deciding where you want to be in that spectrum on any given day.

2. Balance and Expand Body, Mind, and Spirit.

When a person balances their body, there is vitality. When a person balances their mind, they find calmness and ease. When a person balances their spirit, they are able to reach beyond what can be understood in the mind or felt in the body.

When all three parts of us are in harmony, we are able to expand and reach new heights in all aspects of our being. This is a seemingly impossible task, and even if we can achieve it, the effects do not remain forever. Within each human is a vast, ever-changing universe of possibilities, so know that your points of balance are always subject to change.

3. Balance and Expand Self, Partner, and Community.

Everything starts with ourselves. All of our dramas and victories in life stem from our perception. The more balanced we are, the steadier the platform we have to offer others.

We have many partners in life. For me, my older brother was one of my first partners in crime. He taught me how to peel oranges, play with cats, and countless other priceless things. In the years since, I have had many friends, lovers, business partners, and creative collaborators; all have helped me explore who I am by reflecting back to me how I am perceived.

These reflections can sometimes be difficult to digest, even if they are true. In some cases, they may be very distorted. Nevertheless, partnership teaches us a great deal about ourselves and our relationship to the world around us. From there we must decide who we want to be. We must work daily to be that person through our practices. When partnerships are healthy, the collective benefits to humanity are huge.

For the longevity of any relationship, reciprocity—the balance between giving and receiving—is key. The level of reciprocity within a community will largely determine the health and happiness of its members. If you consider yourself a healthy, happy person, the idea of giving love and support to your community becomes a logical next step. Over time it is possible to expand your love to larger and larger groups until you can authentically love all people—i.e., *upeksha, one love, samadhi, nirvana.*

BALANCE PRACTICES

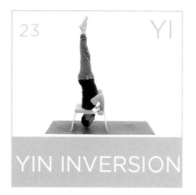

Yin Inversion (YI)

No matter your experience with acrobatics you can play with going upside down and learning to balance your entire body in this new arena.

PROPS NEEDED:
TWO CHAIRS AND A WALL

Place the chairs next to each other, the backs of the chairs touching the wall, with enough space between them to fit your head. If your chairs are hard, fold up a few kitchen towels and place them on the inner edges of the seats, where your shoulders will go.

» Lower your **head between the chairs** to connect your shoulders to the inner edges of the seats.

» With **fingers pointing down** toward the floor, grab the inner legs of the chairs with your hands and **walk your feet in** as close as you can.

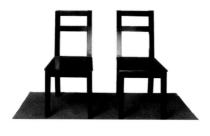

Yin Inversion Chair Set-up

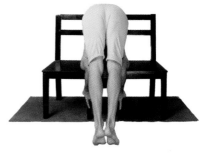

Place Shoulders on Chairs

» While pushing down with your hands, **jump your hips up** and **bend your knees** into a tuck to get upside down.

» Then slowly **extend your legs** vertically. Use the wall to help you find your balance.

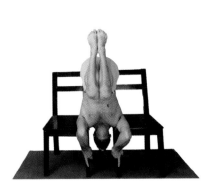

Jump Up and Tuck

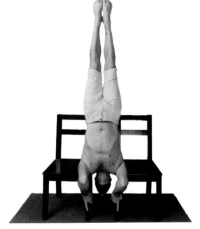

Yin Inversion on Chairs

» Once up, try to **soften your shoulders** to get a nice massage and breathe calmly.

» *When you come down,* ***do a Child's Pose (Ch)*** *for 3–5 breaths to help deepen the benefits of your inversion.*

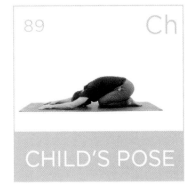

89   Ch

CHILD'S POSE

Train Your Fun Side

Brush your teeth for a week with your non-dominant hand. Working with your "second favorite" side is an amazing practice in patience, slowing down, and appreciating how many years you have done things one way. If you really do this for a week my guess is you will start finding other ways to balance your dominant side with your fun side. Pick any sport, use your non-dominant side, and dig into some awkward yet interesting learning. For advanced students, try a full meal with chopsticks on your fun side!

Zen Rock Balance

This activity has many benefits. Maybe you've been hiking in an enchanted place and you stumble upon a rock balance garden. Depending on the texture, size, and shape of the rocks, you can stack them in a physical expression of static balance. The game consists of you picking a place with rocks, then learning how to spot them, one on top of another, like you spot your friends in inversions. When you line up the angles of the rocks correctly, you will create a unified piece of balanced art.

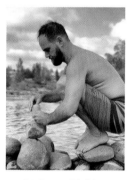

Listen with Your
Eyes and Fingers

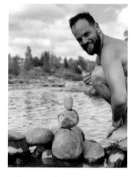

Savor the Moments
of Balance

VISIT **WWW.ACROYOGA.ORG/MCP** TO DOWNLOAD A FREE WORKBOOK, WATCH TUTORIALS, AND FIND OUR COMPANION VIDEO COURSE TO HELP YOU ACTIVATE THE PRINCIPLES AND PRACTICES DISCUSSED IN THIS CHAPTER.

REFLECT & DEVELOP YOUR BALANCE

Balance Journaling is a practice that can unite the harmony of the mind with the balance of the body. The art of training our balance is supported by going into the laboratories of our bodies and measuring where we are and where we want to go. When you are ready to grow your balance, follow this journaling prompt.

Outward Reflection
1. Write the name of someone you know who you think is very balanced.
2. What qualities does this "balanced" person have?

Inward Reflection
3. Where do I have balance and harmony in my life?
4. Where in my life do I want more balance or harmony?
5. What habit, practice, or quality would support the balance of my relationships?

Make a Path Forward
6. What would success look like in my balance-building practice?
7. What skill or move would be a huge milestone for my expression of balance?
8. In pursuit of my balance, what exercises will I dedicate to? For how long?

As an example, your Balance Journaling might look something like this:

1. *Oliver.*
2. *He embodies joy, ease, flow, and steadiness.*
3. *I am balanced between my masculine and feminine sides. I also balance work and play very well.*
4. *I would like more balance between how much I give and receive in general. I would also like to be able to do a 2-minute handstand hold.*
5. *Making more clear boundaries about how much I can give would help my relationships become more balanced.*
6. *Success would look like doing long handstand holds without injuring my elbows.*
7. *A huge milestone for me would be doing a one arm handstand for 30 seconds on each arm.*
8. *Until I can reach my goal of a 2-minute handstand, I will do 3 attempts per week, plus 1 minute of hanging before and after to balance compression in my joints with traction. For my internal balance and relationships I will practice communicating my boundaries more honestly.*

11

SOLAR ELEMENTS AND PRACTICES

This is the bling, the wow factor, and the electrifying part of AcroYoga that will blow your mind again and again. This branch of AcroYoga will help you feel more confident and capable of doing dynamic skills. Learning these elements will empower you and your friends to do things that you might have thought were just for circus freaks!

As you learned in Chapter 2, *acro* means "on the edge" and *yoga* means "union" or "connection," so AcroYoga is the connection found when we go to the edge. Doing acrobatics is a constant practice of being present, aligning with the people you are working with, and finding new edges.

You will face fears, have breakthroughs, and learn a lot about partnership. The teacher is gravity and the practice is about finding the best alignment to make the hard feel easy. There are many potential directions your acrobatic path can take. No matter the direction, the following building blocks will be involved.

FULL BODY POSITIONS AND ACTIONS

These fixed shapes and actions form the foundation for your acrobatic journey. Using this language will support you along your path in AcroYoga by helping you understand, communicate, and execute these essential shapes and movements.

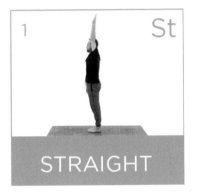

Straight (St)

FOUNDATION: Feet together.

ACTIONS: Reduce any angles in the body until the body is in one straight line.

BENEFITS: Straight is strong; it aligns the bones in order to support large amounts of weight.

CHALLENGES: Nothing about us is made with straight lines. Making our curved bodies perfectly straight is an impossible goal, but one that is worth dedicating to.

DRILLS: Lie on the ground, both faceup and facedown, trying to get the body flush with the floor.

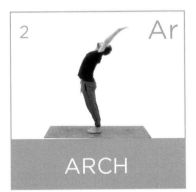

Arch (Ar)

FOUNDATION: Feet together.

ACTIONS: Look up and back, bring hips forward.

BENEFITS: Spinal mobility is good for overall vitality and energy; arching is one of the common positions/actions that creates power in acrobatic and gymnastic movements.

CHALLENGES: Can cause injuries if done incorrectly given the body's strength and flexibility.

DRILLS: Arch-ups: from lying facedown, lift the arms, head, and legs up and away from the floor, then lower back down.

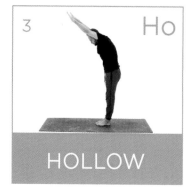

Hollow (Ho)

FOUNDATION: Feet together.

ACTIONS: Pull navel back toward the spine, ribs back toward the spine, and scoop the tailbone.

BENEFITS: Unifies the body; is one of the common positions/actions that creates power in acrobatic and gymnastic movements.

CHALLENGES: Hollow is based on muscular training versus bone structure, so it is harder to learn the optimal hollow shape and more difficult to repeat with consistency.

DRILLS: Hollow-body rocks: from lying on your back in a hollow body position, rock from hips to shoulders.

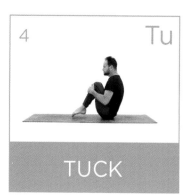

Tuck (Tu)

FOUNDATION: Sit bones.

ACTIONS: Bend knees to chest, bring feet toward butt.

BENEFITS: Best shape to create rotation, i.e. flipping or inverting; does not require hamstring flexibility.

CHALLENGES: Because the legs are bent, it's harder to keep all muscles engaged.

DRILLS: Tuck-ups: from lying on your back in a hollow-body position, swing your arms past your knees and tuck as fast and tight as possible, then return to hollow. *See Solar Asana Sequence page 161.*

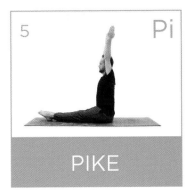

Pike (Pi)

FOUNDATION: Sit bones and back of legs.

ACTIONS: Bring the legs and upper body closer, keeping feet together.

BENEFITS: Increases capacity for rotation, i.e. flipping or inverting, as the legs stay muscularly active.

CHALLENGES: Lack of active flexibility and hamstring flexibility can make this position uncomfortable.

DRILLS: V-ups: from lying on your back in a hollow-body position, keep your legs straight as you lift your legs, arms and chest up as quickly as possible into the tightest V shape you can, then return to hollow.

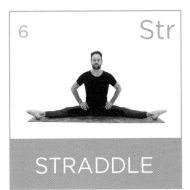

Straddle (Str)

FOUNDATION: Sit bones and backs of legs.

ACTIONS: Separate the feet, keeping the legs active and toes pointed.

BENEFITS: Allows for many L-base flying poses; lowers the center of gravity of the flyer to make poses more stable.

CHALLENGES: Lack of hamstring flexibility can make this position difficult.

DRILLS: Straddle-ups: from lying on your back in a hollow-body position, keep your legs straight and in a wide straddle as you lift your legs, arms and chest up as quickly as possible into the tightest shape you can, then return to hollow.

HAND AND ARM ALIGNMENT

Much of what we do in acrobatics rests on the intelligence of how we align our bones to support our weight and the weight of our partners. Since arms are less powerful than legs, alignment is critical and it is paramount to train the micro angles of the hands, arms, and shoulders.

Each posture in this section offers a different amount of weight to be poured through the arms and hands. This allows us to experiment with little alignment changes in the easier poses before progressing to harder poses that demand better alignment. These micro adjustments are easiest in Table (Ta) Pose and most complicated in Handstand (Hs).

This row in the AcroYoga Table of Elements will help you progressively build toward your handstand. There are other benefits to these poses too, such as opening the hips, legs, and shoulders, but I selected these specifically to prepare you for handstand and partner acrobatic arm balances.

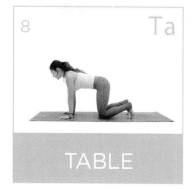

Table (Ta)

FOUNDATION: Hands shoulder width apart, knees hip width apart, feet flexed.

ACTIONS: Align arm bones—shoulders, elbows, and wrists—in straight vertical lines.

BENEFITS: Very stable and easy for all people; a good way to align hands and arms for handstands.

CHALLENGES: Knees on the floor is not comfortable for all people.

DRILLS: Table (Ta) Range of Motion (ROM) for elbows, shoulders, and spine. *See Solar Asana Sequence page 156–157.*

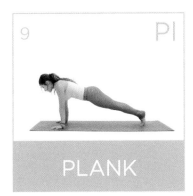

Plank (Pl)

FOUNDATION: Hands shoulder width apart, feet together.

ACTIONS: Unify the body; squeeze elbows toward each other.

BENEFITS: Teaches body unification; is an essential prep pose for Front Plank (FP).

CHALLENGES: Not everyone has enough strength to do this pose.

DRILLS: Tightness drill and push-ups, *See Coaching Plank ATB page 77* and *Solo Strength Practices page 88.*

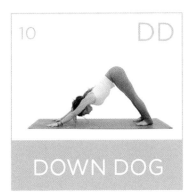

Downward Dog (DD)

FOUNDATION: Hands shoulder width apart, feet hip width.

ACTIONS: Align the body in a straight line from hands to hips; squeeze the elbows in toward each other.

BENEFITS: Trains upper body alignment for handstands with less weight and no fear of falling.

CHALLENGES: Hamstring and shoulder tightness; you can bend the legs and open the hands wider until your mobility increases.

DRILLS: Down Dog push-ups. *See Solar Asana page 160–161.*

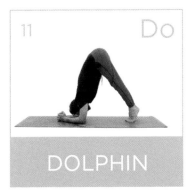

Dolphin (Do)

FOUNDATION: Elbows shoulder width apart, hands interlaced, feet together.

ACTIONS: Align the upper arms as vertically as possible; push down into the floor and hollow ribs toward spine.

BENEFITS: Increases shoulder flexibility; is a great building block for Forearm Stand (4A).

CHALLENGES: Shoulder tightness can make this difficult.

DRILLS: Lift one leg at a time; kick up and switch your legs.

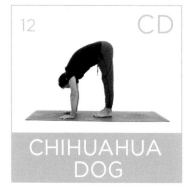

Chihuahua Dog (CD)

FOUNDATION: Hands shoulder width apart, feet together. Arms should be vertical.

ACTIONS: Push down into the floor; hollow ribs toward spine.

BENEFITS: This is the setup for the majority of handstand entries in acrobatics; creates a solid foundation upon which to invert.

CHALLENGES: Lack of hamstring flexibility can limit comfort in this pose; requires awareness of straight, vertical arm lines.

DRILLS: Lift one leg at a time; kick up and switch your legs.

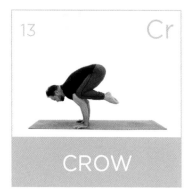

Crow (Cr)

FOUNDATION: Fingers spread wide, hands wider than shoulder width, equal weight on all four corners of each palm. Arms bent, knees resting on elbows or triceps.

ACTIONS: Balance full bodyweight on your hands by pushing through your fingers.

BENEFITS: Teaches fingers how to balance a handstand.

CHALLENGES: Requires core and arm strength; you can't use your hands if you fall out of the pose.

DRILLS: Crow Range of Motion (ROM). *See Solar Asana Sequence page 162.*

FOOT AND LEG ALIGNMENT

Legs are your power as a base and your roots as a spotter. Mobility and stability are both keys to being a great base and spotter. Understanding how to use your strongest muscles and how to plant your feet with a straight spine is half the journey here. The other half is learning how to increase your flexibility after you have warmed up your lower body. Bases will find much more ease as their hamstrings open up.

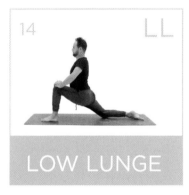

Low Lunge (LL)

FOUNDATION: Front foot facing forward under knee. Back knee, shin, and foot extending back from the hips.

ACTIONS: Bend the front knee; breathe into and open the back thigh and hip.

BENEFITS: Increases hip and leg flexibility.

CHALLENGES: Knee on the floor may be uncomfortable for people with sensitive knees.

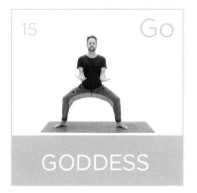

Goddess (Go) aka "Horse Stance"

FOUNDATION: Feet wide, toes turned away from each other, legs bent, heels under knees.

ACTIONS: Ground through the feet with a straight spine.

BENEFITS: Offers variable angles of support for spotting L-base skills; foundational for climbing to standing acrobatics.

CHALLENGES: Requires good balance as it is not stable forward and backward.

DRILLS: Spotter's Dance. *See Solar Asana page 160.*

Warrior 1 (W1)

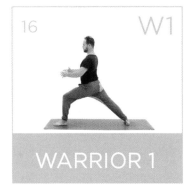

FOUNDATION: Front foot facing forward, aligned directly under front knee. Back foot turned out forty five degrees.

ACTIONS: Bend front knee, ground through the feet with a straight spine.

BENEFITS: Great for spotting skills that move forward and backward.

CHALLENGES: Requires good balance as it is not stable side to side.

DRILLS: Spotter's Dance, Warrior 1 Leg Press. *See Solar Asana Sequence page 160–161.*

Uttanasana (Ut) aka "Standing Forward Fold"

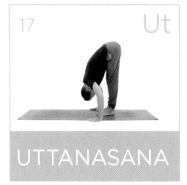

FOUNDATION: Feet together or hip width apart.

ACTIONS: Hinge at hips; ground through the feet and take long, deep, controlled breaths; listen to hamstrings and choose the appropriate variation to find ease.

BENEFITS: Opens the backs of the legs and the entire spine.

CHALLENGES: Tight hamstrings make this pose difficult; pose must be modified depending on flexibility.

VARIATIONS: Feet apart; legs bent; hands on a block. *See Uttanasana (Ut) Flexibility Practice page 104.*

FLEXIBILITY POSES

I think of flexibility like the colors that an artist has to paint with. The more flexible an acrobat has, the more expressive their art can be. For every degree of flexibility you have, you need less effort to do many poses.

As your flexibility increases, the load on your body decreases and the longevity of your practice is supported. This is one of the key principles that many people do not have the patience to train for or to truly understand.

Yogic practices add many layers to traditional flexibility training. Breath and energetic awareness are foundational to how yogic stretching is different from gymnastic stretching. In gymnastics the body is the obstacle; in yoga the body is the teacher. While we open the physical body we can also open subtle energetic channels at the same time to unlock more of our human potential.

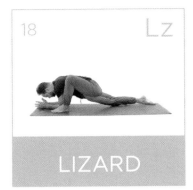

Lizard (Lz)

FOUNDATION: Front foot facing forward, front leg bent. Hands or forearms inside front foot, back leg straight.

ACTIONS: Increase hip range of motion in harmony with the breath; relax muscles.

BENEFITS: Increases hip flexion; helps bases do flying transitions with less effort.

CHALLENGES: Pose must be adjusted depending on flexibility of the hips.

Split (Sp)

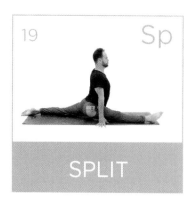

FOUNDATION: Bottom of the front leg, top of the back leg.

ACTIONS: Square your hips and breathe.

BENEFITS: Creates more potential in your movements by increasing your Range of Motion.

CHALLENGES: Leg and hip tightness.

VARIATIONS: Lunge with foot in front of knee; split with blocks under your hands; Half Split (½ Sp). *See Solar Asana Sequence page 162.*

Center Split (CSp)

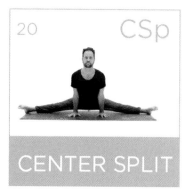

FOUNDATION: Heels.

ACTIONS: Straddle straight legs wide.

BENEFITS: Creates more potential in your movements by increasing range of motion; specifically helps press handstands.

CHALLENGES: Leg and hip tightness.

VARIATIONS: Frog; pancake; supine straddle against a wall; *kurmasana* (tortoise pose).

Wheel (Wh)

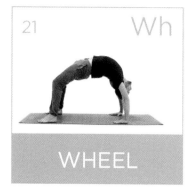

FOUNDATION: Hands shoulder width apart by your head, feet hip width apart and parallel.

ACTIONS: Push into floor to open the shoulders and spine while grounding through the feet and legs.

BENEFITS: Gives lots of energy, opens the shoulders, back, and hips; creates new movement potential.

CHALLENGES: Back and shoulder tightness.

SOLAR ASANA SEQUENCE

The sequence on the following pages brings the solar and yoga elements from the AcroYoga Table of Elements into a practice that you can easily follow along with. After practicing this sequence of *yoga asanas*, or physical postures, you will have a stronger ability to connect the dots of your own body and mind.

As you learn to listen and align your own muscles and bones, you can then apply this wisdom to how you align with others in partner acrobatics. The Solar Asana Sequence is designed to warm the body up and get you ready to train handstands and other acrobatics.

The following sequence contains:

1. **Strength elements:** Bodyweight calisthenics that get easier as your strength-to-weight ratio and technique improve.

2. **Poses to refine your alignment:** Before you stack somebody's weight on top of your hands or feet, become familiar with your most optimal alignment by pouring your own bodyweight through your bones.

3. **Flexibility poses:** The more flexible you are, the more ease you will have in life and in doing partner acrobatics. These poses are hand selected to offer you the ranges of motion needed to help your AcroYoga practice take flight.

4. **Balance poses:** Balance is an essential element in partner acrobatics. To increase the potential for ease and success, each individual should build their own understanding of how to balance by experimenting with their body and gravity.

To follow the sequences on the following pages, move across the pages before starting the next row.

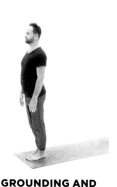

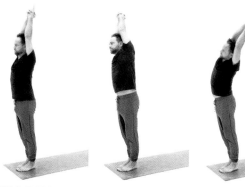

GROUNDING AND CENTERING

Mountain Pose: Feet together, arms by your side, *3 breaths*

FULL BODY WARM-UP

Straight (St): Arms up, fingers interlaced with index extended

Side Bend: Stretch to the right, *3 breaths*

Side Bend: Stretch to the left, *3 breaths*

Back Bend: Look back, arms up by ears, *3 breaths*

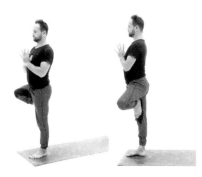

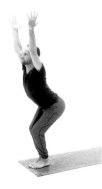

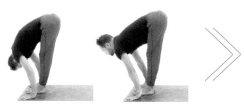

TREE POSE

Right foot up to meet left thigh, hands in prayer, *3 breaths*. Left foot up to meet right thigh, *3 breaths*

CHAIR POSE

Feet together, bend legs, arms up, *3 breaths*

UTTANASANA (Ut) FORWARD FOLD & LIFT

Feet together or apart, legs straight or bent. Relax torso over legs, *3 breaths*. Inhale lift spine halfway, look up

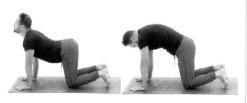

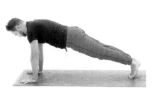

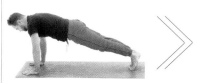

(Ta) SPINE (ROM)

Inhale look up to Arch (Ar), relax shoulders. Exhale look at belly to Hollow (Ho), extend shoulders. *Repeat 2 times*

PLANK (Pl)

Step feet back, feet hip width, arms straight, *1 breath*

(Pl) ELBOW (ROM)

Inhale bend elbows out to the side. Exhale straighten arms and squeeze elbows in. *Repeat 2 times*

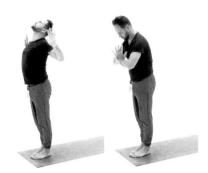

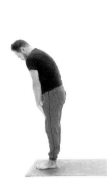

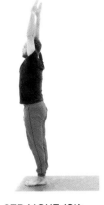

ARCH (Ar) & HOLLOW (Ho)

Inhale open arms to cactus, Arch (Ar). Exhale gaze down, hands in prayer, Hollow (Ho). *Repeat 3 times*

BACK PLANK (BP)

Exhale hands to thighs, squeeze midline, *1 breath*

STRAIGHT (St)

Inhale arms up while keeping ribs in and down, *1 breath*

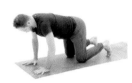

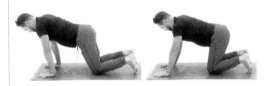

ARM & SPINE ALIGNMENT

Table (Ta): Exhale hands to floor, shoulder width. Step knees to floor

TABLE (Ta) ELBOW RANGE OF MOTION

Inhale bend elbows out to the side. Exhale straighten arms and squeeze elbows in. *Repeat 2 times*

(Ta) SHOULDER RANGE OF MOTION (ROM)

Inhale planche shoulders forward. Exhale open shoulders backward. *Repeat 2 times*

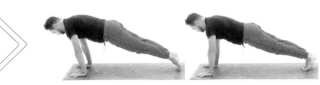

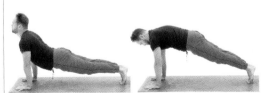

(Pl) SHOULDER (ROM)

Inhale planche shoulders forward. Exhale open shoulders backward. *Repeat 2 times*

(Pl) SPINE (ROM)

Inhale look up to Arch (Ar), relax shoulders. Exhale look at belly to Hollow (Ho), extend shoulders. *Repeat 2 times*

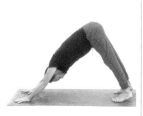

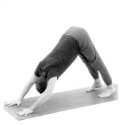

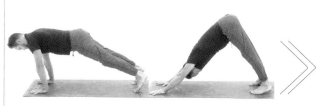

DOWN DOG (DD)

Push hips up and back to Down Dog (DD), *1 breath*

(DD) ELBOW (ROM)

Inhale bend elbows out to the side. Exhale straighten arms and squeeze elbows in. *Repeat 2 times*

(DD) SHOULDER (ROM)

Inhale planche shoulders forward. Exhale open shoulders backward. *Repeat 2 times*

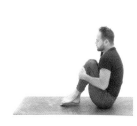

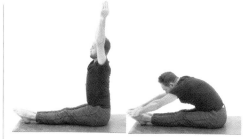

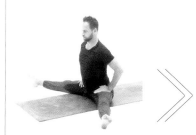

TUCK (Tu)

Pull knees to chest, bring feet to butt, *3 breaths*

PIKE (Pi)

Straighten legs, feet together, arms up, *3 breaths*

Hands toward toes, relax head over legs, *3 breaths*

PIKED STRADDLE (PiStr)

Legs straight, feet as wide as possible, *3 breaths*

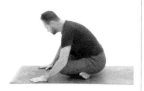

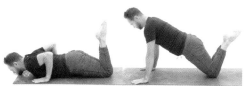

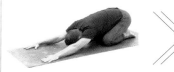

UPPER BODY STRENGTH & MOBILITY

Cross legs, sit up and roll forward to lay chest down

KNEE PUSH-UPS

Prep: Hands wider than shoulders, knees bent, feet together

Straighten and bend arms, keeping body in a straight line, *3–7 push-ups*

CHILD'S POSE (Ch)

Sit hips back onto heels, extend arms forward and relax, *3 breaths*

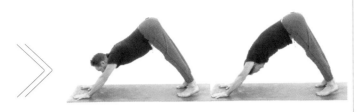 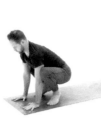 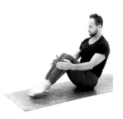

(DD) SPINE (ROM)

Inhale look up to Arch (Ar), relax shoulders. Exhale look at belly to Hollow (Ho), extend shoulders. *Repeat 2 times*

SUPPORTED SQUAT (Sq)

Walk feet forward, bend knees, hands to floor, *3 breaths*

LEG POSITIONS

Shift to seated

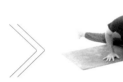 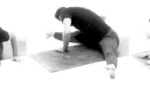 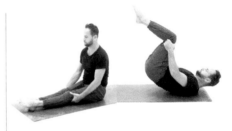

Side Bend: Bring head toward left knee, *3 breaths*

Side Bend: Bring head toward right knee, *3 breaths*

Forward Bend: Hands forward, relax head toward floor, *3 breaths*

TUCK (Tu) ROCKS

Raise torso, bring feet together for Pike (Pi), *3 breaths*

Roll back and forth with knees bent, core engaged, *3-7 rocks*

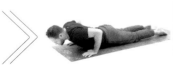 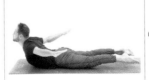 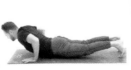 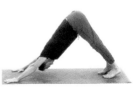

COBRA

Hands in Push-up Prep, inhale lift torso and look up, *3 breaths*

FRONT BIRD (FB)

Lift arms out and back. Inhale look up, lift chest and legs, *3 breaths*

TRANSITION

Push hips up and back to Down Dog

DOWN DOG (DD)

Ground and center, *3 breaths*

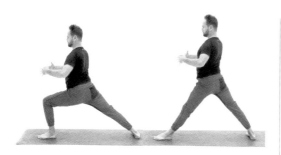

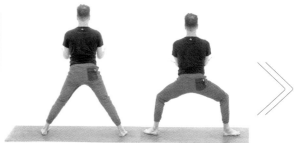

SPOTTER'S DANCE

Step left leg forward. With straight spine, inhale to bend front leg

Exhale to straighten front leg. *Repeat 3 times*

GODDESS (Go) SQUATS

Turn to the right. Stand with feet wide and spine straight

Inhale to bend legs, exhale to straighten. *Repeat 3 times*

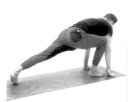

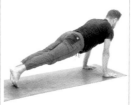

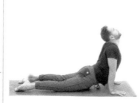

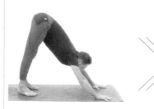

UPPER BODY STRENGTH & FLEXIBILITY

Hands to floor, exhale step back to Plank (Pl)

PLANK (Pl)

Hands shoulder width, arms straight, feet together, *3 breaths*

UP DOG

Inhale look up to Arch (Ar)

DOWN DOG (DD) PUSH-UPS

Walk feet one-third of distance toward hands

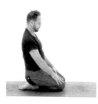

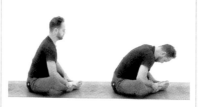

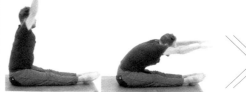

CORE STRENGTH & INVERSIONS

Hero (He) Pose: Sit hips down onto heels

BUTTERFLY (Bu)

Bring feet forward, soles of feet touching, knees open to the side

Hold ankles, bend forward, relax head over legs, *3 breaths*

HOLLOW PIKE (HoPi)

Straighten legs, inhale arms up, look toward toes

Arms forward, exhale ribs in and down, shoulders touching ears

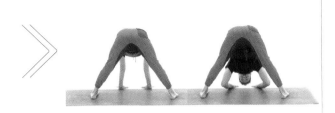

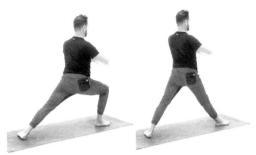

STANDING PIKED STRADDLE (PiStr)

Hands to the floor, spine straight, arms straight

Bend arms, exhale relax head toward floor, *3 breaths*

WARRIOR ONE (W1) LEG PRESS

Quarter turn to the right. With straight spine, inhale to bend front leg

Exhale to straighten front leg. *Repeat 3 times*

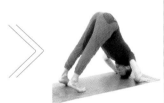

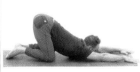

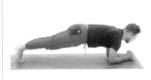

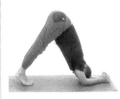

Bend arms, elbows out to the side. Straighten arms, elbows squeeze in, *3–7 push-ups*

ANAHATASANA

Knees to floor, lower chest down, arms straight and thighs vertical, *3 breaths*

FOREARM (4A) PLANK (Pl)

Fingers interlaced, feet together, shift shoulders over elbows, *3 breaths*

DOLPHIN (Do)

Walk feet forward until shoulders are over elbows, look to feet, *3 breaths*

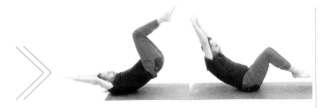

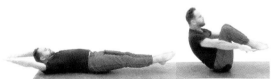

TUCK (Tu) ROCKS

Roll back and forth with knees bent and arms overhead. Keep core engaged, *3–7 rocks*

TUCK (Tu) UPS

Begin in Hollow (Ho)—heels and shoulders off the ground, arms overhead. Exhale to swing arms forward, tuck knees to chest and feet to butt. Inhale to extend back to Hollow, *3–7 tuck-ups*

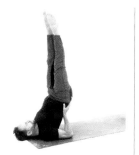

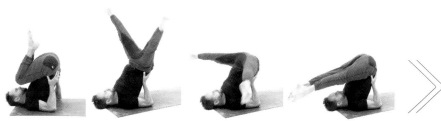

SHOULDERSTAND (Sh)

Roll up to shoulders, legs vertical, hands supporting lower back, *3 breaths*

SHOULDERSTAND (Sh) LEG POSITIONS

Tuck (Tu): Tuck knees to chest, *1 breath*

Open Straddle (OStr): Extend legs to vertical, feet wide, *1 breath*

Piked Straddle (PiStr): Pike legs to floor, feet wide, *1 breath*

Pike (Pi): Bring feet together, *1 breath*

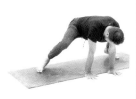

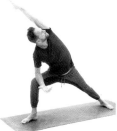

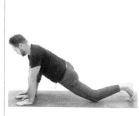

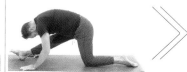

SKANDASANA

Holding ankles, bend one leg, then straighten it and bend other leg. *Shift side to side 3 times*

EXTENDED SIDE ANGLE

Bend right leg, extend left arm in line with left leg, *3 breaths*

LIZARD (Lz)

Lower hands or forearms to floor, left knee to floor, *3 breaths*

HALF SPLIT (1/2Sp)

Straighen front leg, shift hips back, relax head over front leg, *3 breaths*

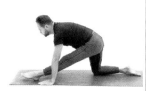

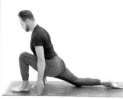

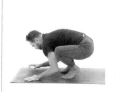

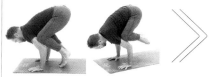

HALF SPLIT (1/2Sp)

Straighen front leg, shift hips back, relax head over front leg, *3 breaths*

LUNGE (Lu)

Bend front knee, hips forward, chest up, *3 breaths*

HANDSTAND (HS) TRAINING

Supported Squat: Step back foot forward, feet wide, knees bent, hands on floor, *3 breaths*

CROW (Cr) WITH (ROM)

Hands wider than shoulders, knees on triceps, lean forward onto hands, lift feet, *3 breaths.* *(ROM):* Lean head toward floor, then back to vertical

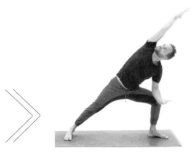

HIP OPENING

Roll forward to feet, step right foot back, bend left leg, extend right arm in line with right leg, *3 breaths*

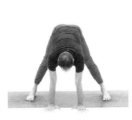

STANDING (PiStr)

Hands to the floor under shoulders, arms straight, feet wide, *3 breaths*

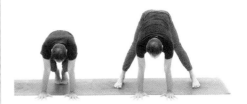

STRADDLE JUMPING JACKS

With hands on floor, jump feet together, then apart, landing softly. *Repeat 3–7 times*

LUNGE (Lu)

Bend front knee, hips forward, chest up, *3 breaths*

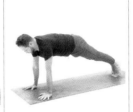

PLANK (Pl)

Exhale step front foot back, feet together, *1 breath*

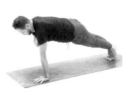

SHOULDER TAPS

Tap opposite shoulder while squeezing all muscles tightly, *7 taps, alternating*

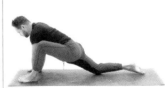

LIZARD (Lz)

Lower hands or forearms to floor, step left leg forward, right knee to floor, *3 breaths*

CHIHUAHUA DOG (CD)

Lower feet, hands directly under shoulders, arms straight, *1 breath*

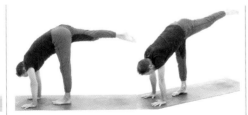

(CD) SPLIT

Lift right leg toward vertical, *3 breaths*. Switch legs, *3 breaths*

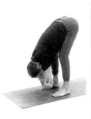

CLOSING GRATITUDE

Fold forward, hands hold elbows, knees bent. You did it! *3 breaths*

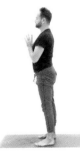

TADASANA (MOUNTAIN POSE)

Stand up, feet together, hands in prayer sealing your practice, *3 breaths*

ACROYOGA ELEMENTS OF FLIGHT

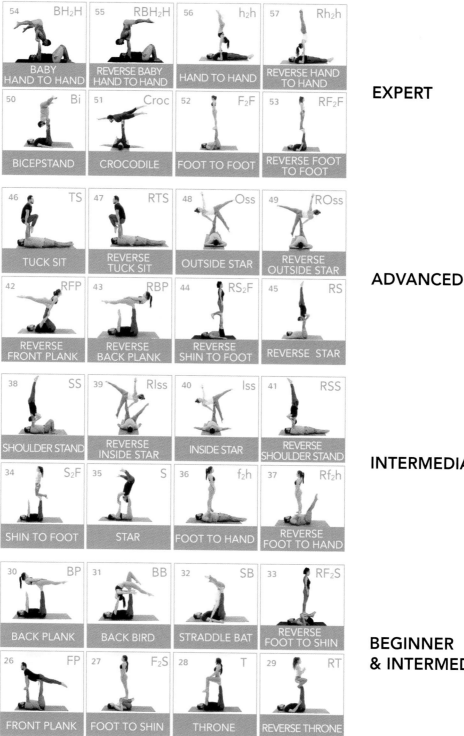

54 BH₂H **BABY HAND TO HAND**	55 RBH₂H **REVERSE BABY HAND TO HAND**	56 h₂h **HAND TO HAND**	57 Rh₂h **REVERSE HAND TO HAND**	**EXPERT**
50 Bi **BICEPSTAND**	51 Croc **CROCODILE**	52 F₂F **FOOT TO FOOT**	53 RF₂F **REVERSE FOOT TO FOOT**	
46 TS **TUCK SIT**	47 RTS **REVERSE TUCK SIT**	48 Oss **OUTSIDE STAR**	49 ROss **REVERSE OUTSIDE STAR**	**ADVANCED**
42 RFP **REVERSE FRONT PLANK**	43 RBP **REVERSE BACK PLANK**	44 RS₂F **REVERSE SHIN TO FOOT**	45 RS **REVERSE STAR**	
38 SS **SHOULDER STAND**	39 RIss **REVERSE INSIDE STAR**	40 Iss **INSIDE STAR**	41 RSS **REVERSE SHOULDER STAND**	**INTERMEDIATE**
34 S₂F **SHIN TO FOOT**	35 S **STAR**	36 f₂h **FOOT TO HAND**	37 Rf₂h **REVERSE FOOT TO HAND**	
30 BP **BACK PLANK**	31 BB **BACK BIRD**	32 SB **STRADDLE BAT**	33 RF₂S **REVERSE FOOT TO SHIN**	**BEGINNER & INTERMEDIATE**
26 FP **FRONT PLANK**	27 F₂S **FOOT TO SHIN**	28 T **THRONE**	29 RT **REVERSE THRONE**	

L-BASE TRAINING

L-basing is when a base lies on their back and presents their legs vertically for the flyer, making an L-shape with their body. There are many benefits to L-base acrobatics: The flyer is close to the ground, so the consequences of falling are less severe than in standing acrobatics. It is easy to get into and out of L-base skills, so you can more reasonably do lots of repetitions in one practice. Because the base is not on their feet and cannot move, it demands the refinement of small details to be stable. Spotting is key to the success and safe progression of L-base training.

ELEMENTS OF FLIGHT

The AcroYoga Table of Elements on page 60 distills the 32 most essential acrobatic poses and organizes them in a logical sequence from beginner to expert based on their technical difficulty and potential danger. They are presented again here so you can see the levels more clearly. Once you master the beginning poses, from Front Plank (FP) to Reverse Foot to Shin (RF2S), you will be able to jam and play with people from around the world! This is by no means a complete list of flying poses, but with each row comes more potential and possibility. Every new skill you unlock further opens the door to a rich journey of self improvement, giggling, falling, trusting, and succeeding.

RANGE OF MOTION (ROM)

There are three steps to Range of Motion (ROM) and this recipe can be used in all AcroYoga poses to expand your collective movement potential. First, the flyer finds ways to move as the base stays stable. If the base is not stable enough the skill will fail, and it will be clear that the base needs to generate more stability in relation to the flyer's expression of movement. Next, the base moves as the flyer stays in one shape. Here the base can remove points of contact, bend, swivel, and expand their mobility and control. The final part of ROM is when both the base and flyer move at the same time. By training Range of Motion this way, you will be prepping for flying transitions and eventually more advanced acrobatic expressions.

BASICS OF SPOTTING

1. **Keep a straight and upright spine when you spot:**
   This supports your own safety and stability. To do this your
   feet should be wide, in a Goddess (Go) stance.

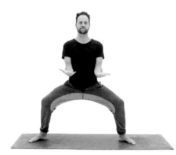

Goddess Spotting Stance

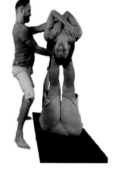

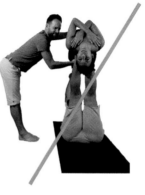

2. **Spot most skills from the side:**
   From the side you can see the base's alignment and support the flyer's safety.

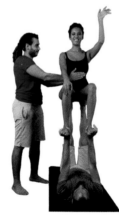

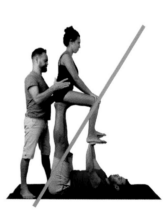

3. **Face your belly toward what you are spotting:**
   Spotters are more stable and powerful when they are centered and facing what they are spotting.

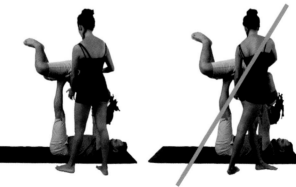

4. **Stay with the center of gravity of the flyer:**
   If the flyer falls, a spotter will be most effective if they are aligned with the center of gravity of the flyer. This is physics and it is standard. There are exceptions, but in general this is where spotters will be most successful.

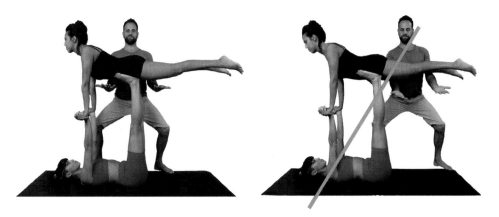

5. **Do the minimum:**
   Sometimes this may mean lifting the flyer's entire body weight. But typically, when the base and flyer have less interference from the spotter they can have a better connection. Like in airplanes, most of the risk is during takeoff and landing, so be ready for both.

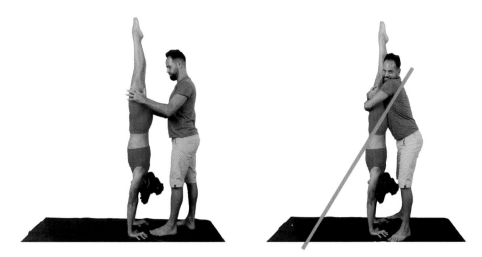

ELEMENTS OF FLIGHT

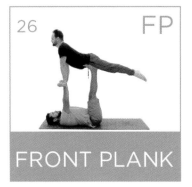

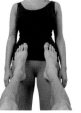 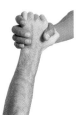

Base's Feet
at Flyer's
Hips

Grip from
Flyer's Point
of View

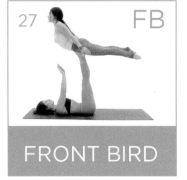

Front Plank (FP)

FOUNDATION: Reverse Hand to Hand Grip, base's feet parallel under flyer's hip bones, heels on flyer's thighs, toes above flyer's hip bones.

BASE ACTIONS: Bend arms and legs to receive flyer's weight, then extend arms and legs vertically.

FLYER ACTIONS: Present hands "FFF" (Flyer's Fingers Forward), unify your body, and lean into base's hands and feet.

SPOTTING: From the side in Goddess (Go) Stance, spine straight, one forearm under the flyer's belly, the other under their legs.

BENEFITS: Strengthens flyer's back and serves as the foundation for many flying transitions.

CHALLENGES: Can be difficult if the base has tight hamstrings and/or does not know how to straighten legs vertically.

Front Bird (FB)

FOUNDATION: Base's feet parallel under flyer's hip bones, heels on flyer's thighs, toes above flyer's hip bones.

BASE ACTIONS: Bend arms and legs to receive flyer's weight, then extend legs vertically and point toes to lift flyer's chest.

FLYER ACTIONS: Unify the body, lean into the base's support and look up; ask for more or less toe point from the base as needed for your balance.

SPOTTING: From the side in Goddess (Go) Stance, spine straight, one arm under the flyer's belly, the other under their legs.

BENEFITS: Strengthens flyer's back and serves as the foundation for many flying transitions.

CHALLENGES: Can be difficult if the base has tight hamstrings and/or does not know how to straighten legs vertically.

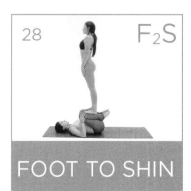

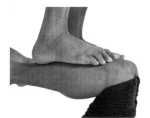

Foot to Shin (F₂S)
Foundation

Foot to Shin (F2S)

FOUNDATION: Flyer's feet parallel on base's shins just below the knee.

BASE ACTIONS: Present hands, draw shins together and keep them sloped up (ankles higher than knees) so flyer's weight stays on the balls of their feet.

FLYER ACTIONS: Connect hands and pour weight through straight, vertical arms; once one foot is in place, step the second foot up; when stable, disconnect hands and stand up.

SPOTTING: From the side, one hand in front of the flyer's belly, the other behind their back.

BENEFITS: Base does not need hamstring flexibility; base and flyer both strengthen stabilizing muscles.

CHALLENGES: Base needs to keep the flyer's feet either parallel with the floor or heels higher than toes.

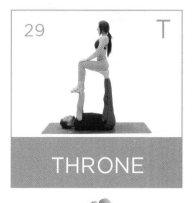

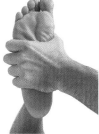

Reverse Foot to Hand
Grip, aka "C-grip"

Throne (T)

FOUNDATION: Reverse Foot to Hand Grip, feet parallel under flyer's sit bones.

BASE ACTIONS: Bend arms and legs to receive the flyer's weight, then extend arms and legs vertically.

FLYER ACTIONS: Standing by the base's head facing away from them, bring their feet to your sit bones and sit onto base's support; once up, bend your knees until your shins are vertical.

SPOTTING: From the side, one hand in front of the flyer's belly, the other behind their back.

BENEFITS: Trains base in deep bending and finding their straight lines with arms and legs.

CHALLENGES: Requires base flexibility to get into the pose; can be difficult if the base has tight hamstrings.

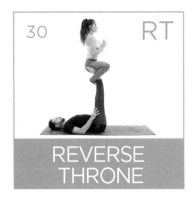

REVERSE THRONE

Reverse Throne (RT)

FOUNDATION: Base's feet parallel outside the flyer's sit bones; flyer's feet hooked around the base's legs.

BASE ACTIONS: Bend legs to receive the flyer's weight, then extend your legs until they are vertical.

FLYER ACTIONS: Stand by the base's hips, facing away from their head; hook one leg around the outside of their shin before jumping back onto the base and wrapping the second leg.

SPOTTING: Same as Throne (T).

BENEFITS: Offers many variations and is a key position for many flying transitions.

CHALLENGES: Hard to get into; base and flyer are not looking at each other so communication can be difficult.

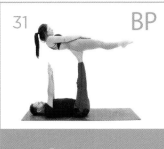

BACK PLANK

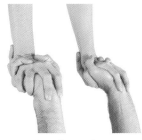

Optional Hand to Hand Grip

Back Plank (BP)

FOUNDATION: Base's feet parallel supporting the flyer's tailbone and lower back. Optional Hand to Hand Grip.

BASE ACTIONS: Flex the feet to invite the flyer, bend arms and legs to receive the flyer's weight, then extend your legs until they are vertical.

FLYER ACTIONS: Stand by the base's hips, facing away from their head, and lean into their support; look toward your toes and unify your whole body in a straight line.

SPOTTING: From the side in a Goddess (Go) Stance, spine straight.

BENEFITS: Unifies and strengthens the flyer; does not require flexibility in the flyer's back; teaches the base to scoop from the heels to get the flyer into the pose.

CHALLENGES: Flyer can fall back onto the base quickly; requires flyer strength to stay in the pose.

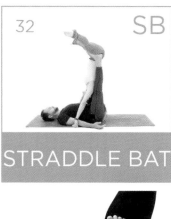

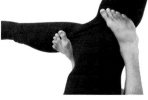

Straddle Bat (SB)
Foundation

Straddle Bat (SB)

FOUNDATION: Feet supporting tops of flyer's thighs.

BASE ACTIONS: From Back Leaf (see page 276), support flyer's shoulders as they bring their legs into position; then adjust feet and keep the legs straight and vertical.

FLYER ACTIONS: From Back Leaf (BL), hold base's ankles, lean back, then maintain your Piked Straddle (PiStr) shape so the base can support you with their feet.

SPOTTING: From the back, hands by the flyer's hips.

BENEFITS: Important pose in many transitions as it is very stable due to low center of gravity and multiple contact points.

CHALLENGES: Base's feet can slide if they are not close to flyer's hip or if flyer cannot keep their Piked Straddle shape.

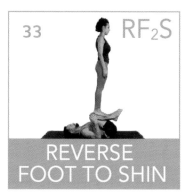

Reverse Foot to Shin (RF2S)

FOUNDATION: Flyer's feet parallel on the base's shins, base's feet at or below their knee level.

BASE ACTIONS: Offer straight arms as flyer steps up; then use your hands to squeeze your legs in. Keep flyer's foot angle steady by not changing your shin angle.

FLYER ACTIONS: Take a Hand to Hand Grip and step one foot at a time; then squeeze your feet toward each other gently.

SPOTTING: From the side in a Goddess (Go) Stance.

BENEFITS: Allows the flyer to control their balance.

CHALLENGES: Can wobble a lot in the beginning; base and flyer are not looking at each other so communication can be difficult.

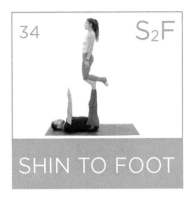

Shin to Foot (S2F)

FOUNDATION: Flyer's shins on base's feet.

BASE ACTIONS: Flex the feet to invite the flyer, bend arms and legs to receive the flyer's weight, then extend your legs until they are vertical.

FLYER ACTIONS: Lean into the base's arms, tuck knees into chest and pour weight into knees. Once the base is stable you can release hands and stand up on your shins.

SPOTTING: From the side in a Goddess (Go) Stance.

BENEFITS: Teaches the base to balance a skill with a high center of gravity; teaches the flyer to trust.

CHALLENGES: Flyer can fall fast and in many different directions.

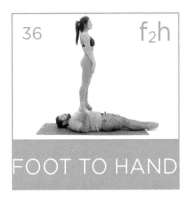

Foot to Hand (f2h)

FOUNDATION: Base's hands over elbows, knuckles of index and middle fingers wrapped around the flyer's heels, palms as big and open as possible, other fingers in contact with sides of flyer's feet.

BASE ACTIONS: Offer feet for support as flyer steps in; then maintain vertical forearms; communicate where the flyer can lean weight for both of you to have more ease.

FLYER ACTIONS: Holding base's feet for support, step into their hands; then slightly point toes, fix your shape, and make subtle shifts considering base's needs.

SPOTTING: From the side in a Goddess (Go) Stance, spine straight.

BENEFITS: Trains the base's grip and forearm alignment for Hand to Hand.

CHALLENGES: Flyer needs to trust base as they are not in control of dismount; can cause wrist compression for the base.

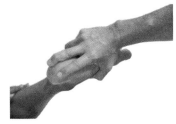

Foot to Hand Grip

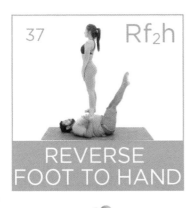

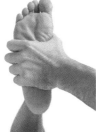

Reverse Foot to Hand
Grip, aka "C-grip"

Reverse Foot to Hand (Rf2h)

FOUNDATION: Base's hands over elbows, Reverse Foot to Hand Grip (also known as C-grip), palms as big and open as possible, making contact with the middles of the flyer's feet.

BASE ACTIONS: From Throne (T) (see page 169), bend and lower arms to the floor; then maintain vertical forearms; communicate where the flyer can lean their weight for both of you to have more ease. To come out, replace feet as flyer sits back to Throne (T).

FLYER ACTIONS: From throne (T), stand up as base bends arms; then slightly flex the feet or keep feet flat, fix your shape, and make subtle shifts considering your base's needs. To come out, sit back to Throne (T).

SPOTTING: From the side in a Goddess (Go) Stance, spine straight.

BENEFITS: Trains the base's grip and forearm alignment for Reverse Hand to Hand.

CHALLENGES: Flyer needs to trust the base as they are not in control of their dismount; can cause wrist compression for the base.

STANDING ACROBATICS

This is where L-base acrobatics can evolve once there is enough trust, experience, and skill developed as individuals and partners. You may have seen these skills from cheerleading or in the movie *Dirty Dancing*. One of the benefits of standing acrobatics is that the base has more mobility. And because standing acrobatics brings people to the edge of what they think is possible, the flyer will often make funny faces and noises as they attempt a skill for the first time!

At this level there is more risk so there is more reward. It is key to have well-trained spotters to make this quantum leap in AcroYoga. When things are not aligned, standing acrobatics can be the source of the biggest and most life-threatening injuries. But when everything is in place, this aspect of the practice can be one of the most joyful and exciting.

Half High

» **Base stands in a Goddess (Go) Stance** with arms bent, palms facing the sky, fingers at eye level.
» Flyer stands close behind the base, taking a Hand to Hand Grip and stepping **one foot on the base's thigh** as close to the hip as possible.
» Base firms all their muscles to **create a solid foundation as flyer steps** the second foot to the base's other thigh. The flyer can push down on the base's arms for extra support.
» Both partners can **free the arms once standing**. To dismount, take a Hand to Hand Grip and step down one foot at a time.

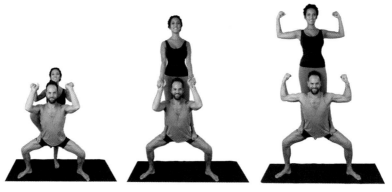

Half High Prep   Half High   Free Half High

Thighstand Counterbalance

For this skill, the base can sit in a chair or do it free (unsupported).

» Base begins with **feet hip width apart** and knees bent. Base and flyer **take a forearm grip** with flyer's palms down, base's palms up.
» Flyer places one **foot on the base's mid-thigh**, turned out.
» Base signals the timing for the mount with an inhale and moving the arms out, then up. Flyer **follows the base's timing, stepping up** onto the base's second leg as they push down into the base's forearms.
» Once the flyer is standing vertically on the base's legs, both then **lean away from each other until arms are straight** to create the counterbalance. The spotter will be at the flyer's back, doing the minimum.

SUPPORTED VARIATION:

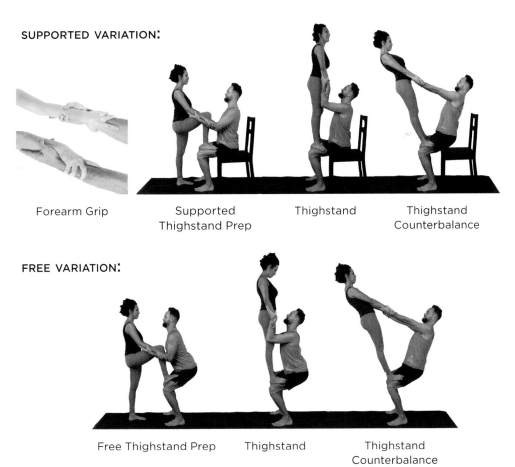

| Forearm Grip | Supported Thighstand Prep | Thighstand | Thighstand Counterbalance |

FREE VARIATION:

| Free Thighstand Prep | Thighstand | Thighstand Counterbalance |

Mono Limb Thighstand

This is the same as the thighstand counterbalance but it starts with the arms crossed. Once you are in the counterbalance you can release one arm and twist away from each other, then switch sides and twist the other way. The spotter will be at the flyer's back, doing the minimum.

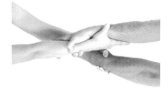

Crossed Forearm Grip

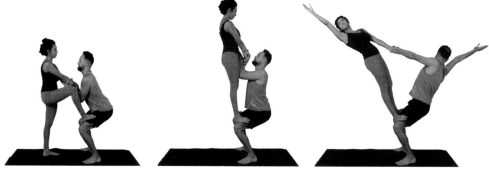

Thighstand Prep   Thighstand   Mono Thighstand
Counterbalance

Split Counterbalance

» **Flyer squats deeply** in front of base, facing away with arms raised vertically.
» Base comes into a squat with feet hip width apart and **base's knees touching**.
» Flyer reaches up and around the base's torso, **clasping their hands**, wrists, or forearms, depending on the size of the base and the length of the flyer's arms.

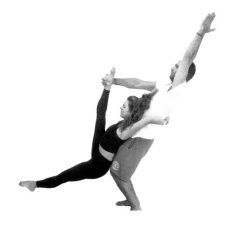

» Flyer **lifts one leg as they lay back** onto the support of the base's knees.
» **Base holds the lifted ankle** of the flyer, then the flyer lifts and extends their second leg. Flyer must move slowly so the base can maintain the counterbalance by matching the amount of lean.

PART IV

MORE FRIENDS, MORE FUN

I think we can all agree that more fun in the world is a good thing, and that having more friends makes the world a happier place. This section of *Move, Connect, Play* offers tools for understanding and grounding your emotions and relationships.

Step one is understanding your thoughts and feelings. Step two is learning to listen to others' thoughts and feelings. Step three is learning to ask clearly for what you want and need, and understanding how to offer the same courtesy to your partners.

The physical manifestation of these practices are partner yoga stretches, inversions, and coaching. Inverting will literally and figuratively turn your world upside down, helping you face fears and build trust with your partners as you progress.

12

EMOTIONAL INTELLIGENCE

The secret of happiness is variety, but the secret of variety, like the secret of all spices, is knowing when to use it.
—DANIEL GILBERT

Emotions are the human spice cabinet; we have developed them in ways that few other species have. Since humans began to write, we have been attempting to describe the complexities of the human condition with varying degrees of success. One of the first books to make mention of human emotions was *The Book of Rites,* a first-century Chinese encyclopedia that identifies seven "feelings of men": joy, anger, sadness, fear, love, disliking, and liking. More recently, Dr. Paul Ekman, a psychologist at University of California, San Francisco, identified six basic emotions (anger, disgust, fear, happiness, sadness, and surprise) and has since launched the *Atlas of Emotions* in partnership with his daughter Dr. Eve Ekman and His Holiness the Dalai Lama. This interactive online platform seeks to help people understand their emotional landscape in order to create a calmer mind. In the following chapter, I will share my own personal atlas with you, as well as the tricks I have learned for navigating the complexities of human emotions in life and in AcroYoga.

The brain is like the conductor of a symphony. There are many musicians in the orchestra playing different instruments, each one contributing to the overarching tone of your life. Some of the instruments in your orchestra include problem-solving, reasoning, communication, listening, and emoting. All of these parts of you are wildly different in how they function and relate outwardly. Problem-solving might require mathematics, reasoning might call for observation and past memories, communication involves language or subtle expressions, and emotions are like waves that move huge amounts of energy through the body.

Anyone who has ever been in love, felt heartbreak, been attacked, or been saved knows that emotions offer us access to great powers that can bring the body into extreme states. It's hard to say what the language of emotions is, but it's easy to say that deep, fully present listening is a great way to help unpack the mysteries behind it. If you are going to listen and offer support to someone, you should try to clarify which section of the orchestra is playing. As our ability to listen increases, our emotional intelligence can become a huge aid in affirming our life and our connections to others.

WHAT ARE EMOTIONS?

The word "emotion" comes from the Old French *emouvoir,* meaning "to stir up," and from the Latin *emovere,* "to move out, remove, or agitate." To survive and thrive, our ancestors needed to empathize with one another in order to make collective decisions that would support the group. Emotions are one of our guidance systems that helps us evaluate if we are in alignment with our goals and desires in life. When we think of a basic emotion such as joy, we can create a simple picture in our minds of what that might look like. But under that seemingly simple emotion is a complex dance between the brain and the body. In the brain, the limbic system is the center of our emotional universe, and is made up of many structures including the amygdala, hippocampus, and basal ganglia. As the hub for all things emotional, the limbic system helps shape our experience of the world and how emotions play into our idea of self. It also regulates endocrine function in response to emotional stimuli. Together your brain and body serve as the bartender for your thirsty soul, serving up chemical cocktails which include:

ENDOCANNABINOIDS: the "bliss" molecule
DOPAMINE: the "reward" molecule
OXYTOCIN: the "bonding" molecule
ENDORPHINS: the "pain-killing" molecule
GABA: the "anti-anxiety" molecule
SEROTONIN: the "confidence" molecule
ADRENALINE: the "energy" molecule

While this is far from a complete list, these are the primary neurotransmitters sparked when doing AcroYoga. The mind has been studied thoroughly and there are countless data sets explaining its intricacies, but the spirit is harder to explain and even more so to define. According to Traditional Chinese Medicine, the emotional layer lies between the spirit and mind and is housed in different organs. The heart relates to joy, spleen to worry, liver to anger, kidney to fear, lungs to sadness and grief, and so on. As much as we love to isolate things in order to understand them, we are byproducts of our thoughts *and* our emotions. Posing one of the greatest paradoxes in science, a photon acts as both a particle and a wave. How can something be two different things? There are many layers to reality, and the same can be said of our consciousness.

Listening to our emotions means learning who we are and what moves and stirs us, what sparks joy and what creates suffering. We are wired to have these emotive states to bond with others and to create boundaries. Emotions are oftentimes not logical, but the more you understand their tremendous power and potential wisdom, the more you understand yourself. In order to understand your emotions, you first have to feel them.

LEARN TO FEEL

Children are incredible teachers of how to feel and express emotions. Suppression of emotions is a learned behavior usually developed as a coping mechanism, especially in response to external expectations placed on us such as "big boys don't cry." Some of us have gotten so good at emotional suppression that we don't feel much at all anymore. If we do feel our emotions, we can't possibly understand where they are coming from. Finding physical and emotional safety can help redevelop our sensitivity and ability to feel again.

As you go through the physical poses in the AcroYoga Table of Elements you will find new emotional edges and attempt harder, riskier skills. Fear, frustration, joy, elation, confidence, and loads of high fives are in your future. This practice will help you to feel many emotions that might have been lying dormant. Once they show their faces, it is possible to go deeper into the mystery and origins of those feelings. From this place of understanding, you will have more success connecting to others and potentially supporting their emotional states too.

ACCEPTANCE

It's okay to feel whatever it is we feel.
—FRED ROGERS

You don't have to understand in order to accept. Rather, accepting is a doorway to understanding. How deeply do you feel? Do you have the courage to express what you feel? Once you connect to your feelings, a next step can be to find ways to express your emotions safely, productively, and honestly. This is key to creating your ideal AcroYoga training environment. Accept that you still have fear and want a spotter. Accept that you are frustrated that your hamstrings are stiff and L-basing is not easy for you. The opposite of acceptance is fighting, suppressing, ignoring, or hiding. These reactions create a time bomb in your relationships and your emotional body. Having emotional intelligence means allowing yourself to be

okay with your emotions and not letting others steer or change your emotional compass.

REACTING VERSUS RELATING

Reacting and relating have many letters in common, but their meanings are quite distinct. The distinction lies in having the sensibility to pair the ideal emotion with any given event. Your partner says, "Why are you so afraid of doing a standing Hand to Hand?" You can react by getting defensive and saying, "You try it and we'll see how brave you are!" Or you can say, in a grounded and confident tone, "I saw a flyer get injured doing that skill so I want to go through the progressions and have spotters that I trust for my first few tries."

Emotionally reacting keeps someone at arm's length from your wounds. It protects your vulnerable spots. Conversely, relating brings someone close in the aim of helping them see and feel your perspective more clearly. Reacting is rooted in fear while relating is an act of lowering your guard to foster trust and compassion. You most likely will never have full control over your emotions; life would be pretty boring if you did! But as you find freedom from your knee-jerk emotional reactions, you gain the ability to relate to a situation or a person from a place of self-awareness and to communicate with a tone which might serve you and the situation better—using the right spice for the right dish.

BOUNDARIES VERSUS BARRIERS

Setting boundaries creates freedom because it removes the uncertainty of the question, "How close do I want to be?" Boundaries are consciously expressed limits that are supportive for co-creating a safe collaborative space, which in turn allows for more exploration. It is key when we do partner work to know that we all have boundaries and we all have the right to shift these from more protective to more open, or vice versa, at any time. From this container of clearly stated boundaries, partners can grow as they know the "rules of engagement."

In contrast, barriers are often not consciously placed—they are like scar tissue. They form around a wound for protection and can sometimes end up stagnating the body, emotions, and relationships. Barriers create distance and separation where boundaries can invite people closer by creating a clear container. Boundaries are expansive, proactive steps whereas barriers are limiting, reactionary steps. In AcroYoga, someone saying, "I will do the skill, but only if we are on good mats with a spotter," is a boundary, while saying, "I won't do it, I'm too scared," is a barrier with little room to move forward. In touch and massage, saying, "I am sensitive with touch around my chest; please work on my upper body but skip my chest," is a boundary, whereas "Don't touch me there!" is a barrier.

There are times when boundaries are supportive and times when barriers are more appropriate. If you generally want to invite more connection, but also avoid certain types of connection, this is a recipe for boundaries. If you do not want to expand or grow your connection for any reason, throw up a strong barrier. How do we understand if we are creating boundaries or barriers? We need to know our triggers and our emotional wounds, and how they block or build our potential in relationships.

LEARN YOUR TRIGGERS

In AA they always say to you, "How come your family knows how to push your buttons? Because they installed them."
—ELIZABETH GILBERT

Your family may not have created all of your emotional wounds, but they sure have the potential to rip the bandages off of them. Though we have access to many emotional states in any given moment, we each have our own default reactions—the instantaneous emotional responses we experience time and again in stressful or challenging situations. We all have different types of physical and emotional wounds that originate from our childhood, our relationships, our work environment, or any situation where we experienced a strong negative emotion or sensation. We have an evolutionary advantage over many other animals in that we remember and record these events so we can avoid them in the future. Sometimes our recording system is too good and we store these wounds far longer than they serve us.

Triggers are like sticks of dynamite set to blow when people or situations ignite an explosive response within us. Learning where your pain comes from and what triggers you is a huge asset in the quest to being able to balance your emotional states. The more you know about these parts of yourself, the more clearly you can communicate about them, helping to create an environment where your partners can support you with sensitivity and awareness.

In Buddhism, there is a parable that likens suffering to being hit by an arrow. The Buddha once asked a student, "If a person is struck by an arrow, is it painful?" The student replied, "It is." The Buddha asked again, "If the person is struck by a second arrow, is it even more painful?" The student replied again, "It is." The Buddha then explained, "In life, we cannot always control the first arrow. However, the second arrow is our reaction to the first. And with this second arrow comes the possibility of choice." While we can't control our outside environment, we can, with practice, avoid being shot by the second arrow. There are two very effective exercises that you can practice in order to circumvent this human response to life. First, be aware of the pattern of the second arrow, and second, practice kindness to yourself when you see it coming.

Every training partner I have had the pleasure to work with has taught me so much. Each partner requires a different set of circumstances physically and emotionally to thrive. Sometimes I get it "right," while other times I miss the mark completely. Take this story, for example: Humor is one of the ingredients I cherish in my training. I love to make fun of myself, my partners, and life as I train. One day I was asking my partner if she remembered the corrections from our last practice of a specific skill. She looked at me with a blank stare, big eyes, and smiled at me. I said, "You have the memory of a goldfish." We both laughed and kept training. A few weeks later she had the courage to share with me that when she was growing up she had dyslexia and other learning disabilities and thought she was stupid. When I said she was like a goldfish, she felt deeply hurt because I had found a trigger. My arrow hit that older wound, but of course I did not want to hurt her. She was my partner and I wanted only the best for her. I apologized, she forgave, and we established a new boundary that ensured we would both feel happy and safe while training.

Silly comments are meant to make us laugh and bring us closer together. Sometimes they work, sometimes they backfire. We agreed not to defend our position when the other is sharing their emotions, but to listen to how the other

feels. We committed to assuming the best intent of the other, knowing we wanted to keep humor alive in our training. We knew that practicing with little or no emotion was not an option for either of us, so these new boundaries would be a way for us to keep our spiciness alive and allow for moments of realignment when we discovered an emotional edge.

To heal your wounds, you can work on accepting where you are emotionally and committing to doing the daily work needed to release your pain, learn from it, and stack up new, positive experiences going forward.

YOUR HAPPY PLACE

Along with movement, I have spent countless hours refining my taste for the yummy things in life. One of my very happy places involves putting on some Bossa Nova music, opening a nice bottle of pinot noir, and cooking a delicious meal for people I love. I know this about myself, so I make a point of doing it often. In your acro partnerships, know what you like and what your partners like, and be sure to include those things in your training. It's a simple recipe, and often the ingredients of success (in

AcroYoga as in life) are not difficult in theory. The tough part comes in the execution. If you have new skills you're trying to learn in addition to a training program you need to get through, can you also find time to incorporate your partner's favorite skill? Or add on a few therapeutic moves at the end of a long, grueling session?

In the long term, if we cultivate positivity and joy, our achievements will add up and we will stay motivated to continue the endless journey of AcroYoga. Prioritize making space for the fun, easy, and yummy stuff—once there are enough pieces of your life moving in a positive direction, the critical mass takes over. By establishing your happy place and visiting it often, you can expect an increase in your emotional stability.

EMOTIONAL BALANCE

Your emotions are meant to fluctuate, just like your blood pressure is meant to fluctuate. It's a system that's supposed to move back and forth, between happy and unhappy. That's how the system guides you through the world.
—DANIEL GILBERT

Emotional balance does not imply that you will not suffer, feel sadness, or have only happy dances. Rather balance is the ability to accept the emotions we feel in any given situation, thereby empowering ourselves to embody the wholeness of who we truly are. The more we are in balance with our emotions, the more happiness we can experience and share with others because we are aware, full, centered, and accepting in who we are.

And there will come a time when differences no longer harass you.
—YOGA SUTRAS OF PATAÑJALI, 2.48
TRANSLATED BY GESHE MICHAEL ROACH

In 2020, Black Lives Matter became a global movement denouncing the systemic racism that has been part of the fabric of American society since its inception. Racism is one of the byproducts of differences harassing us. Practicing tolerance and acceptance of yourself and others is a powerful way to measure your success in emotional intelligence and it is a clear path toward more global unity.

If at an AcroYoga class you are instructed to go look for a partner, the monkey mind can take over. Some people will immediately think, "Who is the cutest, smallest, strongest, funniest, best-smelling person in the room?" Others might think in terms of negatives: "I don't want to work with beginners or people who've never tried this skill." The phrase *never judge a book by its cover* has proven true time and time again. Often, our "book cover" perceptions can lead us to untruths. Our greatest victories in AcroYoga can often come from the people who we least suspected would get us there. The more centered we are, the less we cling to what we think we want, or run from what we think we don't want.

NOBLE ELEMENTS OF THE EMOTIONS

These three Noble Elements are like emotional keys; any one of them can be enough to unlock stuck emotion. As you learn to mix all three, you can become an emotional alchemist and create positive environments where emotional expression feels natural and easy for those around you.

Fun (Fn)

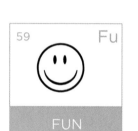

Laughter is the shortest distance between two people.
—VICTOR BORGE

There are times to be serious, there are times to have fun, and there are times to have serious amounts of fun. Fun is the "why" of AcroYoga. All people enjoy fun. It makes life worth living. The extremes that fun dances between are happy and sad. There are moments for both emotions and fun can be the catalyst that brings you from one end to the other. If you are sad and you have fun, you might become happier. If you are happy and things unexpectedly lose the fun factor, you might become sad.

Your emotional body is directly connected to your endocrine system, which is your personal pharmacy that floods your blood with feel-good chemicals. You get an adrenaline rush when you take risks in acrobatics. You then get further rewarded by a dopamine fix when you perceive that you "did the skill right." All of these actions and biochemical reactions spark states of enjoyment, amusement and pleasure. As AcroYogis, we welcome fun into our practice, our relationships, and our life. My advice: *Play more!*

Support (Su)

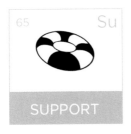

By the time we reach adulthood, most people have felt at some point as if they were mentally sinking. At such times, the support of others can literally be a lifesaver. To physically do AcroYoga we must give and receive support, just as in order to live we must breathe. Support is the breath of the practice: when things are working properly, it comes in and out seamlessly and consistently.

Support is key to our existence and exists on the spectrum between independence and dependence. Sometimes being independent and self-supporting serves you better, while at other times your dependence upon others can empower a friend or partner to step up and throw you the life ring you needed. Support in one another sparks co-creation—one of the fundamental pillars of AcroYoga.

Connection (Cn)

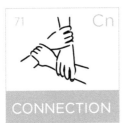

All sentient beings developed through natural selection in such a way that pleasant sensations serve as their guide, and especially the pleasure derived from sociability and from loving our families.
—CHARLES DARWIN

The Noble Element of Connection is depicted by a base, flyer, and spotter holding one another. Three is the smallest number of people needed to create a community. In traditional yoga, we first learn to connect to ourselves. Next, we have the opportunity to test our yogic theories in our relationships and partnerships. We might believe we are patient until we are tested by our partners' needs or desires. The unique challenges of partnership can help us see our strengths and weaknesses. We bond with the help of oxytocin; when it is present in our bloodstream, we trust more and give more. Our AcroYoga practice causes our brains to release this addictive chemical, and as a result we can build a huge family of playful movement monkeys. Our connections can expand exponentially, from three to thirty to three hundred!

It is also key to regularly connect with yourself, especially the deeper you go in relationship with others. Closeness and space are the two sides of the connection coin. Both sides play a role in building healthy connections. I am sure AcroYoga would not be a global practice if it were not for the fact that one of the best byproducts of doing AcroYoga is the community that forms around it. When activities are fun and there is support, people will become connected—there is no way around this truth!

"Happiness is when what you think, what you say, and what you do are in harmony."

—MAHATMA GANDHI

EMOTIONAL INTELLIGENCE PRINCIPLES

1. Celebrate First, Refine Second.

It is common to finish some AcroYoga skills and have a list of five things you did not like about your attempt. If as partners you learn to start by sharing one positive thing first, you become more open to receiving each other's feedback. Positive is good. Specific is better. "You did a great job," doesn't let your partner know why it was great, whereas "You did a great job moving slower," is specific.

From that emotionally affirming place, you can refine one thing to keep moving in the direction of progress, both emotionally and physically. This is one of the most important shifts in training that makes you an AcroYogi versus a skill-chasing acrobat.

As a way of relating to the skill and to your partner, celebrating first and refining second improves the quality of your connection and therefore your collaboration. You are making investments in each other's emotional bank accounts and improving your combined technical awareness at the same time.

2. Love Heals.

Love is an impossible word to define, but humans will always pursue the impossible! Just like yoga, love has many layers, styles, and definitions.

In Buddhism there are four aspects of true love:
1. *Metta*: loving-kindness
2. *Karuna*: compassion, the ability to support others who are suffering
3. *Mudita*: sympathetic joy, the happiness for others' happiness
4. *Upeksha*: equanimity

The Ancient Greeks classified love in eight ways:
1. *Eros*: sexual passion
2. *Philia*: deep friendship
3. *Ludus*: playful love
4. *Agape*: love for everyone
5. *Storge*: love for family
6. *Pragma*: long-standing love
7. *Mania*: obsessive love
8. *Philautia*: love of the self

Like our bodies, our emotional fabric can be wounded, injured, and develop scars. In the process of healing, we often experience a wide array of emotions. When I get injured, my most common reactions in progression are: disbelief, anger, frustration, sadness, despair, surrender, curiosity, acceptance, and eventually integration and healing.

Through each injury, we can gain physical skills, emotional tools, and life-altering gems of wisdom. You might learn new training techniques with one hand as you heal a wrist; you may learn a meditation technique to help process your emotional states. In every wound there is potential for growth.

To heal is to make something more whole, and this does not require you to have "MD" after your name, years of professional training, or other accolades. One of the most powerful aspects of healing is love, because of how profoundly it moves us. Much of healing is just that—being able to move what is stuck.

Mixing the brilliance of our minds with our emotions creates an even stronger healing potential. A surgeon who looks at your file on a clipboard, takes off her gloves, holds your hand and tells you, "You are in good hands," is the miracle of integrating emotional intelligence with Western medicine. When someone looks us in the eyes and shows up with any of these elements of love, they can melt many blockages in the body, priming the soil of our being for deeper transformation.

3. Ask for What You Need.

This may sound simple, but for many of us it is scary. It requires both courage and humility. When everyone in your community of three asks for what they need it keeps the practice safe—physically and emotionally.

In this collaborative, nurturing environment, progress happens faster and with less drama. Often this principle takes the form of setting boundaries. Sometimes it's more about invitations. No matter the direction of the conversation, the practice of asking for what you need will get you and your partners talking about how to set up ideal conditions to reach your individual and shared goals.

Some of us may pride ourselves on our ability to endure suboptimal conditions. A more sustainable approach to training is learning to co-create the optimal environment for you and your partner's growth. To do this we practice speaking up—clearly, compassionately, and often.

4. "No" Is a Complete Sentence.

We do not always understand our own emotions, nor do we need to in order to honor them. This applies to others too. It is not necessary for others to understand our emotions in order to respect our boundaries. To have a safe community, consent is vital and revocable at any time with the powerful two-letter word, "no."

All people know how to say "no"; for many babies, it's their first word. But many of us lose the power to say no in certain scenarios, especially when we feel scared or pressured. Remembering that we have a right to say no at any time is crucial to feeling heard and respected, and to expanding our potential for collaboration and connection.

If others do not have the capacity to respect our simple "no," they are not yet worthy of our interaction, our trust, or the privilege of building an AcroYoga practice.

"It's not about how much you do, but how much love you put into what you do that counts."

—MOTHER TERESA

EMOTIONAL INTELLIGENCE PRACTICES

Pink Pill or Blue Pill?

One of my dear friends, Nayef Zarrour, offered this pearl of wisdom to me years ago: He told me that when his girlfriend would share a problem with him, he would ask if she wanted the pink pill or the blue pill. The pink pill was to hold space for her and just listen. The blue pill was to offer thoughts, insights, and feedback.

Usually when he would share his problems with me, I would ask if he wanted the purple pill—a blend of listening, holding space, and offering potential solutions. To know how to support others, the first step is to identify what aspect of support they need and what support looks like for them.

Pink Pill Practice

Find a friend and for five minutes straight, practice just listening. This does not mean you cannot say any words; you can still speak. The difference is, any words you use should affirm what they are saying or be in service of them sharing more.

Here are some examples of affirmations:

» *"Yes"*
» *"Right"*
» *"I see"*
» *"I hear you"*
» *"Tell me more"*

Blue Pill Practice

Find a friend and for five minutes, practice listening just like you did in the Pink Pill exercise. After listening, share some reflections you have about the situation at hand—thoughts, insights, and feedback. Remember, you are proposing ideas for how they might refresh their perspective. It is not your job to fix their problems, rather this exercise is an opportunity to bring new light, and ideally new questions, to the conversation. Take this example:

Topic: *My partner gets mad when I feel scared of doing new skills.*

Blue Pill responses:

» *"That kind of takes the fun out of new skills, right? Have you told her how you feel? Maybe she could fly more to get a taste of fear. Then her compassion and understanding might grow."*

» *"Bummer, sorry to hear that. Have you both aligned around what goals and qualities you want to grow in your partnership? It's up to both of you to speak your needs, hear each other, and make agreements about how you want to train."*

Humans are like onions—we have lots of layers and sometimes, we induce tears. This practice is one of many ways to develop your capacity to ask good questions, listen deeply, and learn to offer the right kind of support to someone in need.

VISIT *WWW.ACROYOGA.ORG/MCP* TO DOWNLOAD A FREE WORKBOOK, WATCH TUTORIALS, AND FIND OUR COMPANION VIDEO COURSE TO HELP YOU ACTIVATE THE PRINCIPLES AND PRACTICES DISCUSSED IN THIS CHAPTER.

13

THE YOGA OF RELATIONSHIPS

God, grant me the serenity to accept the things I cannot change, the courage to change the things I can, and the wisdom to know the difference.
—THE SERENITY PRAYER, REINHOLD NIEBUHR

It is in our relationships with others that our true nature is tested. As enlightened as we may be in our meditations, our relationships reveal where we really are in our journey of self-knowledge, confidence, trust, and communication. We might think we are very generous until someone asks for our favorite toy, and in that moment we see our true nature. Relationships, be they romantic, platonic or otherwise, expand our human potential beyond what we can accomplish alone.

My mom dropped a wisdom bomb on me years ago about relationships when she shared this story: A friend asked her to write down the top five things she hated about my stepdad. My mom was delighted by the opportunity to vent. She made the list and could not wait for her friend to hear the top five ways

her husband made her life difficult. When they saw each other, her friend asked, "You got the list?" My mom replied, "You bet I do." Her friend asked, "And you want more harmony in your relationship?" "Sounds divine!" said my mom. "Rip up the list and accept who he is," her friend replied. "Have the confidence that you can keep living your life, he can live his life, and you can accept each other as is." Learning that we cannot, with any degree of certainty, change other people's minds or behaviors, but that we can only change our own minds and behaviors, was a revelation I'll never forget.

It must have been a tough pill to swallow, but she ultimately thought it was a valuable enough lesson to share it with me. Tossing out our list of frustrations with our partners—or our "wish lists" of all the things we'd like them to change or become—does not mean we can't share our feelings and ideas with our partners about how the relationship can be improved. It does, however, encourage us to refocus our attention and energy on elements of the relationship that we *can* control—our ideas and attitudes. If we base the success of our relationships on how much we can change others to fit our desires, not only are we likely to be disappointed, but we miss out on the opportunity for the personal growth and development that is unlocked by true healthy partnership.

In this chapter, I want to share what I have learned in the many partnerships I have had over the past thirty years. I have had acrobatic partners, coaches, co-founders, co-teachers, business partners, and lovers in my journey. The many things you have read in this book were written in many different environments: on the road during my gypsy days when I had many friends and adventures; in Santa Monica where I had an amazing, dedicated, high-level acrobatic partner and my first stable home after my gypsy years; and most recently while self-quarantining during the COVID-19 pandemic with my partner in crime in Mexico. The insights

in this section have been tested in my own personal practice during some of the most intense cohabitation conditions I have experienced. It has taken a lifetime to arrive at the clarity I have on how I do and don't want to relate to others. There is still a lifetime of learning ahead, but here is what I have already learned: When I look at my life and where I have invested most of my time, energy, and love, it has been in my relationships. Yoga gave me a clear template—be nice (*ahimsa,* or non-violence) and don't lie (*satya,* or non-lying).

In his work with marriage and family counseling, author and speaker Gary Chapman offers us the *Five Love Languages*: words of affirmation, acts of service, quality time, gift giving, and physical touch. It is common to give the kind of love that we like to receive, but our partners might crave a different kind. It takes time, communication, and receptivity to be good at the partner game. You have to *want* to get better to excel in partnership—it does not happen by accident.

An inescapable truth is that we as humans cannot live without the support of others. Especially now as our society becomes more and more compartmentalized, we are all part of a massive market where we each invest our time training in a specialty and performing one or a few specific skills. This market allows us to live without having to grow and cook all our own food, design the chips and program the code in our smartphones, or build the cars we drive to work. We lean into so many people we will never meet. These angels are labeled as strangers not to be trusted or considered friends. How we think about and relate to these people is core to our worldview. Practicing AcroYoga with many "strangers" can help us see that we are all connected and our fate as a species is supported when we acknowledge that. One might say that relating to others is one of the most valuable skills we can develop as humans.

What I decided many years ago is that I want to be friends with everyone I interact with. Whether it's my mother, lover, accountant, or a stranger, they all get the same handshake of kindness and honesty from me. Although some people will be closer than others, I've simplified how I want to primarily relate to all people, and that is through friendship. If I start there, I believe all the other hats we might wear will be supported by our base of friendship. We can be friends with the milkman, the nurse, the auto mechanic, the farmer, the tax man, etc. Sometimes in business it slows things down, as you have to address emotions and other aspects of your connection that take time to align. Still, the benefits are huge, especially when things are not going well. In fact, there was one year when my accountant did my taxes for free because he knew I did not have the money and because we were invested in each other as friends. Our relationships with one another are not trivial parts of our lives; they are fundamental and essential to our wellness. As we exchange the currency of trust in our relationships, we gain courage and deeper self-knowledge.

WAYS OF RELATING

Truth Is the Way

As truthfulness (*satya*) is achieved, the fruits of actions naturally result according to the will of the yogi.
—*YOGA SUTRAS OF PATAÑJALI*, 2.32
TRANSLATED BY GESHE MICHAEL ROACH

Lying is the fastest way to erode trust. There can be many short-term gains from lying, but if you look at the long run of your life and your relationships, honesty (and, if you want really strong relationships, brutal honesty) is key. Sharing the truth is not always easy, but it should always be valued and prioritized. This *sutra* says that when true honesty is achieved, your thoughts, words, and actions will flow naturally. Your will becomes your reality. If you don't believe this, try being completely truthful for a week and pay attention to the shifts in your mental and emotional states, as well as the quality of your connections with others.

Assume Best Intent

We were all raised by different people and gifted different tools for relating to others. If someone acts in a way that you don't like, you have choices. You can take offense and raise your defenses, you can ignore and suppress your reaction, or you can become curious and assume they are doing the best they can with the tools they have. I have observed thousands of AcroYogis in my time, and I cannot say that I have ever seen a flyer deliberately make mistakes to upset their base, or a base who dropped their flyer on purpose. If we assume that we are all doing the best we can with the skills we have and the bodies we were born into, we can create community based on compassion—one where we can lift one another to new heights. Assuming best intent allows people the space to be able to share honestly, without judgment or defensiveness.

Share What You Feel

Even though we cannot rely on changing other people's minds, we can always share with others how we feel. It often takes courage and vulnerability to share what you feel. You might not get the support or response you hoped for. You might fear being judged. There are risks involved, but the cost of not being honest with the people you love outweighs them all.

By sharing what you feel, you give others the opportunity to value your feelings and accommodate your needs. If my partners do not share with me that my foot placement in Star pose is chafing their skin, I will not know I am causing discomfort. Over time all the flyers will run away in fear when they see me coming! A simple question like, "How did that feel for you?" can get a very potent conversation started that helps both partners find more awareness and synergy. The details of how you communicate are another story, but no matter the method of delivery, sharing what you feel is one of the most crucial facets of healthy relationships.

Stay In Your Lane, Don't Blame

When conflict arises we must have the courage to own our contribution to the friction. In relationship, you are either 50 percent of the drama or 50 percent of the solution. Life is short and blame is a waste of precious life force. The ideas of right and wrong are responsible for most of the world's suffering. The world is not black and white; there are many shades of gray. Polarizing and attacking others is not a feasible way forward. When in conflict or disagreement, confidently share your ideas of how to make things better and be open to hearing other perspectives on your behavior and interactions with those involved. Respond versus react, and stay in your lane, meaning know what is your work, and what you can invite from others.

Being Right and Letting Go

Our intellectual capacity is truly amazing, and so too is our ego's desire to be right! Conviction is a big part of human empowerment. This is your third chakra helping you feel and express your power. Also called the *manipura chakra*, this energy center is located at your center of gravity. It is your willpower—what supports your ability to make change in the world. There are people who are deficient in this area and others who have an excess of conviction. The cool thing is that you can be right *and* you can also let go. Warning: I am not encouraging you to be passive aggressive, but quite the opposite. You can have your conviction and not need to convince others of it; that is the letting go part. Whatever is true for you today, chances are it will change over time. When you pair your mind's capacity to know with the emotional wisdom of humility, you allow the space for others to do the same. Being right is a moving target, so letting go will be a lifelong teacher.

Judgment and Separation

Our minds are incredibly effective in evaluating our surroundings and informing us if we are safe. This is exactly what happens when we unconsciously or inadvertently label something as good or bad. Our worldview is in our hands; we can have our own preferences and at the same time we do not need to label the whole world based on our emotional state. If we are late, and we jump in the car and get behind someone who is not in a hurry, or someone cuts us off, what usually happens? We assume the worst about other drivers on the road—they are stupid, selfish, and we hate them! Yet in these snap judgments there is a lot of information missing. Geshe Michael Roach says, "Don't judge people unless you can read their minds." This in itself is powerful, but he continues: "If you could read their minds, you would want to serve them."

If we more clearly understand others, the wounds they have endured in the past, and their present struggles, we can have so much more compassion and empathy for them. If I understood that the driver cutting me off was racing to the local school because they heard their child had been injured, or that the slow driver in front of me got into a car accident last week and is struggling to overcome that trauma, I would be less inclined to jump to conclusions about their behavior. We make these snap judgments because it is easier to put an imaginary barrier between us and someone else than it is to take in the bigger picture. We all want the same basic things in life: to feel loved and supported, to laugh, to eat yummy

food, etc. Knowing how similar we are at the core is a worldview that holds many positive benefits. As beautiful as connection is, for it to be sustainable we have to look at how much we give and receive from the people we are connected to.

Balance Giving and Receiving

I am a recovering over-giver in relationships. I love that about myself; I see the positive effects resulting from the way I have given in the past, and I feel happy with my choices. At the same time, I have another fifty years ahead to live and, God willing, reach my goal of one billion AcroYogis! For me to reach these higher goals in life, I have to play the long game and allow as much support to come in as I put out. In the times that I have over-given, I unknowingly set myself up for my expectations to be let down in my relationships. "I did x, y, and z for you and you did not give back to me."

When giving and receiving are out of balance, you set the relationship up for pain, instability, and drama. If I over-give I can unintentionally create the expectation that my partner needs to give more. If I under-give, the sustainability of our relationship is put in question and insecurities can develop on the receiving end. It takes receptivity to know where you are on the spectrum of giving and receiving. Get to know your tendencies and move toward the middle road to develop more ease and success in your relationships.

Give and Take Space

Anyone who has ever successfully made a campfire knows the importance of space and properly sized wood. A fire needs a spark and the right conditions to become an inferno. If you throw the heavy logs on too early or don't give the fire enough access to oxygen, the fire gets suffocated and dies. Partnerships need the right conditions to grow too. Small sticks and leaves are little topics like, "Do you want to train two or three times per week?" Or, "What types of warm-ups and therapeutics do you like?" The heavy logs are bigger topics like, "Do you want to move to China and study partner trapeze?" or "Do you want to start a hippie commune based on reiki healing, contact improv, and the nutritional value of hemp seeds?" The intensity of the topic has to match the intensity of the fire already present.

Giving space allows your partner to have solo time and the ability to clarify what they want and need as an individual. If your partner is not freely offering you the space you need, you can take a walk, listen to a podcast, or directly tell them that you need space. Honesty is always supportive in the long run even if it is not what the other wants to hear. The fire of transformation is central to relationships. For this fire to work for you, you must learn to tend it correctly.

NOBLE ELEMENTS OF RELATIONSHIPS

Relating is a surefire way to test and refine who we are. These Noble Elements are ingredients in the recipe of getting to know the real you and mixing your essence, your fears, and your dreams with those of others. These elements can be your guides: they will show up strongly when you are relating in a healthy way in your AcroYoga practice, and will spill over into the other realms of your life as well.

Confidence (Cf)

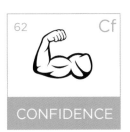

Confidence supports your growth as an acrobat. The more acrobatics you train, the more your confidence will grow. It can be a positive loop that feeds itself when you train in the right conditions. This is true for building confidence in any situation—keep doing the thing you want to get better at.

Confidence and arrogance can sometimes be confused as we learn to step into our acrobatic power. Confidence is an internal sense of self-worth that helps you show up in the world, both for yourself and on behalf of others. By contrast, arrogance is an outward performance of superiority, which often acts as a mask to hide a lack of true confidence.

When you learn to move through the world with confidence, your clarity of mind and your emotional stability will empower you to take hard but necessary actions. As we gain confidence we move from unsure to certain. The best thing a flyer ever hears from their base is, "I got you." That phrase is born out of confidence.

Trust (Tr)

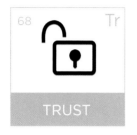

We all have aspects of us that are protected, closed, and trapped. I chose an open lock as the symbol for this Noble Element because when we trust we open up; we unlock ourselves from behind the doors that usually hold us back and we allow ourselves access to new ways of being. Trusting, having faith, risking, and letting go are all pieces of living a more full life. Negative interactions create more protection and fear. Positive interactions feed trust. Trust cannot be demanded, it must be earned. Moving from fear to freedom is a sign that trust is developing.

Self-Knowledge (SK)

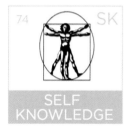

The *Vitruvian Man* was designed by the Renaissance genius Leonardo da Vinci in the fifteenth century. This drawing depicts a man in two superimposed positions with his arms and legs apart and inscribed in a circle and a square. The drawing and accompanying text are sometimes called the *Proportions of Man*. Leonardo dedicated his life to the pursuit of knowledge in numerous fields. He dissected humans and many other animals to understand how the body works.

Self-knowledge is the byproduct of daily embodied research. Self-knowledge grows alongside your ability to look at your life objectively and to make decisions that are in harmony with who you really are. When we ground our true desires and test ourselves in relation to others, we can realize either, "Yes, I am that brave," or "No, I still have lots of fear." On the other side of these experiments we realize more about where our strengths lie and what areas need our attention. On the spectrum of self-knowledge we move from ignorance to wisdom.

The great philosopher Socrates once said, "The unexamined life is not worth living." We have our whole lifetimes to get to know who we are. Ideally over time we come to know more and more of who we are and how we can arrange our lives in a way that honors what we need to be happy.

We are designed to grow, evolve, and change. Each day, we wake up with different biochemistry, from different dreams, with different lists of things we want to do that day. The more we understand our patterns, fears, and desires, the better we can align our lives and then align with others.

RELATIONSHIP PRINCIPLES

1. Be Kind.

The word "kind" comes from the root *kin*, meaning "family." Kindness is an activated form of love. It is a potent, nourishing force of life.

For many of us, daily servings of self-care are easily skipped. We are often our own harshest critics—thinking, saying, and doing mean things to ourselves. We think things like, "I don't know why anyone would want to work with me," or "I suck at basing this skill!" Then we hide in the corner at the acro jam because we have planted the seed that we are not good enough to be accepted as we are.

Our potential to be kind must start with ourselves. Over time we can expand who we offer this kindness to: At first we offer kindness in our closest relationships. Eventually we can extend that kindness to acquaintances, and then strangers.

It's much easier to be kind to others when they are kind to you first. But what about those who hate us? As this practice deepens, you can grow your capacity to love and be kind to everyone—even those who hate you. It is destabilizing in a powerful way to be kind to someone who is treating you poorly.

2. Practice Perfect Fit.

Our bodies were engineered for perfect fit. The golden ratio is a mathematical relationship that describes how perfect fit is embedded in our design. For example, the length of the last three bones in your index finger are such that you can curl your finger into itself like a fern leaf.

How we apply the principle of Perfect Fit to AcroYoga is that we practice arranging ourselves with others in a way that is comfortable for all involved. Our bodies are like puzzle pieces; the better we get at fitting them together, the more potent and easeful our connection becomes.

On a macro level, how you fit your personality, dreams, and quirks with those of the people around you makes even more use of this principle. In relationships, Perfect Fit is the practice of knowing what is important to you and making sure you are balanced in how you and your partner attend to each other's needs.

3. Use "We" Statements.

There are three aspects to any relationship: you, me, and we. This is yet another shift of perspective and word selection. "Can you slow down?" is grammatically correct and gets the key information across. But, "Can *we* slow down?" is also a correct statement and captures the reality that both partners are part of the solution.

This concept can be taken to extremes: "Can we straighten your elbows?" is not correct—that is something that one partner needs to do. With a greater awareness of "we," we can learn to speak to and make asks of our *partnerships*, rather than just of other individuals. The result of this is more cohesion and synergy.

4. Enjoy Mutual Support.

If you want to excel at giving you must learn to receive in a balanced way, as this sustains your capacity to care for others. One ideal to cultivate in partnership is the ability to lean into each other's support at the same time.

Imagine two thirsty souls in the desert with a huge cup and two straws. One person is holding the cup, the other is pouring fresh cold coconut water into it, and they are both drinking at the same time. This is the beauty and potential of mutual support. Both partners are doing different things, but both are winning.

In AcroYoga, as I offer my partner a therapeutic flight, physically I gain strength and flexibility while they receive decompression in their spine. Emotionally I feel happy that I can help them feel good, and they feel happy to be cared for. Any time you give support, the potential is present for mutual support to take place.

RELATIONSHIP PRACTICES

After theorizing about relationships in the first part of this chapter, now we will test the principles with partner yoga. Yoga is about connecting with and expanding who you are. Partner yoga is a practice where both partners improve their listening, communication, and teamwork.

When you tune in to these qualities, your breath will be synchronized, soft, slow, and deep. You will find that your movements will harmonize as a result of your ability to listen deeply and sense the other.

Taking advantage of your partner's body weight, or using their body like a yoga prop, can help you open up and go deeper into postures with less struggle and exertion. Aligning breath and making modifications for more ease and mutual support are all aspects of what you will train and hone in this part of the chapter.

These exercises can be a way to warm up and calibrate, or to cool down and integrate after a session. You will know it is working when your connection and trust improve and your bodies feel better.

Mutual support is the aim and the intention of these practices, and as partners you will both have to be flexible and receptive to each other to reach that collectively supportive place.

Squat Counterbalance

» Take a **crossed forearm grip and squat** down with your partner.

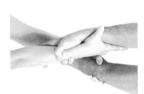

Crossed Forearm
Grip

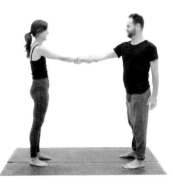

Standing Crossed
Forearm Grip

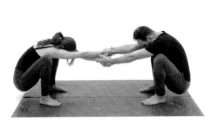

Squat with
Rounded Spine

» **Release your left arms**, keep your right arms connected, and **slowly lean away** from each other until you find straight arms and straight spines.
» You might have to adjust the distance of your feet from each other to find this geometry.

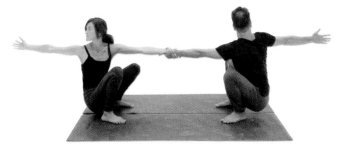

Squat Counterbalance

» Enjoy exploring different stretches and micro tractions. Your **free arm can reach away from your partner** or support your neck as you back bend or do anything that feels good.
» *Stay for 3-5 breaths, then stand up and repeat by releasing the right arm and keeping the left connected.*

Seated Partner Side-Bend

» Start in a **seated Piked Straddle (PiStr)**. If this position is not comfortable, you can sit on a yoga block or pillows until your hamstrings gain more flexibility.

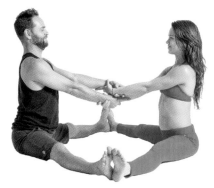

Seated Piked Straddle

» Take a **crossed forearm grip, then release one arm** and reach up and over to opposite sides until you feel a stretch you enjoy.

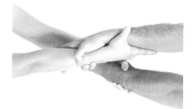

Crossed Forearm Grip

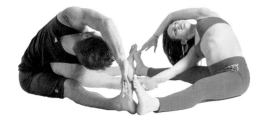

Partner Side-Bend

» The arm that is connected can **pull to create some resistance**, bringing that shoulder closer to your partner.

» *Stay for 3–5 breaths, then repeat on the second side.*

Mini Backpack

>> Start by **standing back to back**.
>> The **flyer bends their knees** enough to fit their mid-back at the base's hips.
>> The flyer then **leans back onto the support of the base** as the base leans forward to create a solid platform for the flyer to open their mid and upper back.
>> *Stay for 3–5 breaths, then switch.*

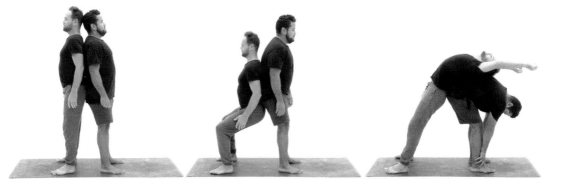

Stand Back to Back   Flyer Bends Knees   Mini Backpack

DOWNLOADING YOUR EXPERIENCE

After partner work it is supervaluable to practice exchanging feedback. I have distilled a simple and effective recipe to gather the wisdom from these physical practices: *Celebrate First, Refine Second.* First both partners share positive feedback—try to be specific. Then both partners share evolutionary feedback—what could evolve to make the experience even better next time.

This ritual helps you invest in each other and build trust and understanding. When both partners are committed to honest feedback and evolution, they can grow together for many years.

14

INVERSIONS AND COACHING

Progress is impossible without change; and those who cannot change their minds cannot change anything.
—GEORGE BERNARD SHAW

Every master of any discipline reached mastery, to some degree, because of a coach. Other than your blood family relationships, the coach/athlete, teacher/student, guru/disciple relationship is one of the oldest and most sacred. Guiding people in inversions is present in all three of the roots of AcroYoga—acrobatics, yoga, and therapeutics. Over thousands of years yogis have distilled the application of inversions for balance and healing properties; acrobats have mastered the most advanced expressions of inversions to push the limits of human biomechanics; and AcroYoga therapists have learned how to fly people in inversions to decompress the spine and restore physical balance.

Seeing the world upside down has many upsides! There are countless benefits and shifts that people experience by

trusting, becoming more empowered, and changing their perspective. Acrobats spend a lot of time refining their skill, control, and strength while they are inverted, as solo inversions are one of the foundational building blocks of acrobatics. Spotting is also an essential part of growing your acrobatic relationships. Before attempting to spot complex partner acrobatics, it is smart to start by learning how to support a single person going upside down on the most stable base ever—the earth! The teamwork developed here will help you unlock many of the more complex flying skills later in your acrobatic journey.

As variable as the universe is, gravity is a steady teacher that can help you understand many things about your body and mind. As AcroYogis learn how to align their bodies with gravity, many impossible things will become second nature. There is a refreshing shift in your mental and emotional state when you invert, and this is why people get hooked on inversions.

WHAT IS AN INVERSION?

An inversion is any physical pose where we have our head below our heart. Downward Dog, Child's Pose, Shoulderstand, Headstand, and Handstand are all examples of inversions.

COACHING

From the beginning of your journey with AcroYoga you will become a spotter, and spotters eventually become coaches. A coach is someone with some experience, an outside perspective, and the desire to help others. With that definition there are countless coaches around us constantly! You have five main tools when coaching: your eyes, your ears, your brain, your words, and your touch. Your eyes see what is right and what can be improved; your ears hear what the athlete is experiencing and feeling; your brain processes the information from your sensory organs and draws conclusions; your words speak to what specifically is going well and what could evolve; and your touch can point out where someone is aligned or misaligned.

Often you have to change your physical perspective to see clearly all the different angles of the body. You also have to know what you are looking for. Humans are wired for seeing the world with a negative bias; this is a vestigial mechanism from our genetic past when we were being eaten by beasts bigger than us, and for survival we needed to see what was wrong and dangerous in our environment. Looking for what is going well requires training, will shift your emotional state, and will give you the ability to strengthen your and your partner's mood and technique. Always celebrate one victory you see in a skill you are coaching before giving a refinement. Be specific, not just nice. Saying, "Oh, that was so good!" makes your AcroYoga partner feel good but teaches them nothing about their technique. Instead try, "Oh, that was so good! *Your arms were straighter.*" This supports their emotions and informs their physical practice.

Your touch can communicate so much. I have had the honor of having quite a few of my masters teach me through touch. My Chinese circus master trainer, Lu Yi, would kick my free hand while training one-arm handstands and say, "You don't even know you have left hand!" But the same man would be so soft and subtle when he spotted my legs in handstand transitions. Touch comes in many forms and magnitudes that all have to find their right place and time.

HOW TO COACH FOUNDATIONS AND ACTIONS

Teaching other teachers has helped me identify what I look for when I am coaching people. I can scan a room of AcroYogis and in ten seconds know what I need to do to maximize my support for the students. I look for two things first off and in this order: the foundation(s) and the action(s).

The foundation of any solo pose is what touches the ground. In a tree pose your standing foot is the foundation. In partner work the contact points between the partners are the foundation. In a Foot to Shin pose, the flyer's foot on the base's shin is the foundation. Everything in AcroYoga and in life starts

with a foundation and is built up or broken down from there. Making sure the foundation is set how you want it is step one. From there it is essential to understand the key actions of the skill being attempted. Action describes what is moving or what muscles are activated to create stability. In golf, the foundation is the hands gripping the club and the action is the golfer's swing. The golf swing has many, many moving parts and different angles, so mastering this "simple" swing takes years.

In training I like to say, "The first three don't count, but don't fail four times." When I say they don't count, I mean that you shouldn't obsess over the first few tries. See if there is a trend after you do three attempts, and from there you will have a reasonable amount of data to create theories about what you can modify. Not failing four times in a row is a good rule on many levels. If you are failing at a skill you are taking a toll on your emotional body and quite possibly your physical body; it is better to take a step back and train a piece of the skill or a more basic form of the skill. Every successful attempt in a practice builds your confidence and the neural pathways in your brain for continued and sustainable success.

When you first learn how to spot

someone it is about safety—more or less keeping them from landing on their face. As your experience grows you can become a magician with how you help others through touch. Listening and asking good questions helps you understand what they feel and don't feel. I remember one day Lu Yi was coaching me, my friend Carolyn Cohen who was a recreational AcroYogi, and a high-level handbalancer. Carolyn put her hands at Master Lu Yi's feet, ready to attempt her first handstand with him, when he said, "Wait, why you do handstand?" She stood up and pondered for a moment or two. Then she replied, "I do handstands because they make me happy." At that moment I saw the power of knowing a student's 'why.' If you don't know their 'why,' you don't know what kind of coaching will get them to where they want to go. Lu Yi was more or less nice to me when I did my attempts. The high-level handbalancer was trying to be a professional performer, and after each attempt he would hardly say a word to her. His subtle and not so subtle body language said something like, "You suck, and you have so much more work to do to reach your high-level goals." But every time Carolyn went, Lu Yi lit up and was so kind to her so he could help her reach

her goal of being happy. I trained with him for five years and cannot express how many lessons he imparted to me. I'll leave you with one of my favorites:

It's not one technique for one hundred students, it's one hundred techniques for one student.
—MASTER LU YI

ARE YOU BREATHING?

One of the first questions I ask someone when I am spotting them in a handstand is, "Are you breathing?" When they don't answer, I know the answer—there is no breath moving at all! Breathing techniques in inversions depend on the type of inversion and your skill level. You don't need to overthink it; if you are breathing and you are upside down that is a victory. If it is an easy inversion for you, you can play with different types of breathing, but in general you want your breath to feel easy and comfortable.

KNOW YOUR ENTRY AND EXIT STRATEGY

Inversions are only good for you if

they are safe. Getting into and out of inversions are the risky parts, so you need to have an idea of how you will navigate these two moments. The exit is actually the first thing you should think about. Ideally you have a spotter to add support and a set of coaching eyes. Your spotter also needs to know how you will go in and out of the pose so they can stay safe. If you kick your spotter because they did not know how you were going to swing your leg to get inverted, they are no longer able to help you and your exit will be like jumping out of a plane with no parachute.

ASSESS YOUR SPOTTER'S SKILLS

At the minimum, a spotter will help your takeoff and landing in your inversions. Once that is in place, maybe they can see different technical things you are or are not doing. It's important to know what you can trust your spotter for. Maybe you are a big human and your spotter is a little human. If you have a lot of fear about your entry and exit, maybe they can be your coach and another bigger person can be your physical spotter.

When you feel safe your inversion practice can be more effective and therapeutic.

HANDSTAND TRAINING

For a great number of reasons people around the world obsess over learning handstands more than almost any other physical pose. Handstands have the potential to help you understand fear, trust, patience, persistence, partnership, and many other aspects vital to the growth of any acrobatic practice. No matter how talented you are, there is always more to learn with handstands and many breakthroughs that happen along the way. These pivotal moments hold meaning unique to the practitioner and their personal journey in acrobatics. Start by believing you might be able to do a handstand. From holding one by yourself for three seconds, to your first attempt at a one-armed handstand, the gifts and refinement of this practice just keep coming.

The foundation of handstands and many skills in acrobatics includes how to align the hands and arms. There are twenty-seven bones in the hand and wrist, and three main bones in the arm. This is why aligning the hands and arms is such an important and detailed job. In general we are looking for straight lines through the arms, as much as the bones and muscles will allow. The less weight, the more precise we can be about micro movements to improve efficiency. Once an alignment is found, it can be challenged by adding weight and holding for longer periods of time. Start with Table (Ta) pose and work your way up with Plank (Pl), Down Dog (DD), Dolphin (Do), and eventually Handstand (HS), gathering information, sensations, and clues to unlock ease in your individual practice.

INVERSION TRAINING PITFALLS

Inverting involves the risk of falling. Our wrists and shoulders were not designed like our ankles and hips were. Our ankles and hips evolved to support our full bodyweight. It's not that our wrists and shoulders cannot take the load of our bodyweight, but depending on your strength, flexibility, and technique, you might put an unintelligent amount of force on a given joint and cause injury.

The most common injuries in acrobatics tend to be overuse injuries because once you get to a certain point in your training, inversions become addictive due to their physical, mental, and emotional benefits. It takes proper training and coaching to expand your capacity for inversions, and each person has a different innate capacity. Knowing and respecting these limits is not always how people practice, and that over-enthusiasm can lead to further imbalances and setbacks.

INVERSIONS AND COACHING PRINCIPLES

1. Train ATB: Alignment, Tightness, Balance

Alignment, tightness, and balance are the foundational trio to every acrobat's practice.

Alignment is the art of using your flexibility and strength to find optimal stacking of your bones. Our bones have genetically evolved to interact with gravity; we can hold a lot of weight for long periods of time as we learn to rely on our bones.

Tightness is the act of squeezing your muscles around the optimal bone alignment. Our muscles are like ropes that can temporarily bind around our bones to make our whole body act as one. Your mind is incredible at computing many complex things simultaneously, and the fewer moving parts in your body the easier it will be for your supercomputing cerebellum to help you find the still point.

Balance is the mystical, magical, even distribution of weight that allows you to stay steady and upright (or upside down), while performing various postures. Balance is much easier to find and maintain when our bodies are aligned and tight. From that place of integrity, the final steps are fixing our gaze on the ground and tapping into the subtle sensations in our foundation.

2. Always Thank Your Spotters.

More than any other principle, this one fans the flames of AcroYoga so strongly because spotters keep the community safe, thriving, and reaching new levels. Without spotters there is no community and there is no practice.

Being a skillful spotter is a game changer in itself because you can be a part of helping someone do something they did not know was possible. Always thank your spotters and grow your community by being that amazing spotter that helps someone feel trust, stay safe, and find success in their inversion.

There are so many people who will support you along your AcroYoga journey. Thanking them is one way to ensure that they feel recognized, and it speaks to the humble fact that we need one another to reach new heights.

3. "Be humble and repeat." —Arno L'Hermitte

Achieving a state of mastery is often done through the accumulation of thousands of small, humble steps. I would not recommend that you set mastery itself as a goal because it is not the desire to reach mastery that brings greatness—it is the dedication to humility and repetition.

4. Remember to Ask, "How did that feel?"

Spotters see and support, but the person doing the inversion feels. When you ask them, "How did that feel?", their answer can help you as a spotter steer your feedback to them.

Maybe I am spotting my friend in what I see as a very weak handstand with hundreds of inefficiencies, and after a few shaky seconds of being inverted they fall to the earth like a sack of potatoes. But when I ask, "How did that feel?" they respond, "That was the best handstand of my life!"

When you coach someone in an inversion you are coaching their body, mind, breath, and emotions. When they come down you become a detective, searching for clues to help you understand where they want to go from where they are in their practice. Don't get lost in the mind; do just enough fact-finding to get back in the laboratory of space and let gravity do most of the teaching.

INVERSION SPOTTING TECHNIQUES

Inversions are one of the most complicated things people attempt and they can be the most transformational. But underneath their glory they are usually supported by spotting. Good spotting is harder to do well than the inversion, yet there is little glory for spotters. As a spotter your role in the community is essential.

Hands On

This is just as it sounds. When a flyer feels the spotter's "hands on," it can be like an emotional blanket of support as much as physical. In inversion training our fears need support as much as our bodies; this technique is the best way to support both, and it is very standard.

Hands On spotting usually means **assisting the flyer at the hips**. The hips are important landmarks on the body for two reasons: First, they are able to take a lot of force; seatbelts are put around this area due to its inherent strength. Second, they are **near the body's center** of gravity; this means that supporting your flyer at the hips **allows you to move their weight with ease** and a very low risk of injury.

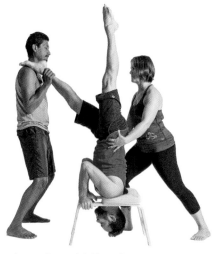

Inversion with Two Spotters

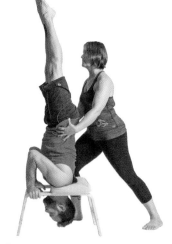

Hands On Spotter Supports the Hips

Scissor-Lift

When you're still **learning to enter an inversion,** whether a shoulderstand or handstand, having the support of Scissor-Lift spotting can help you can **sneak up on it in a slow and** controlled manner. The following steps to a Scissor-Lift will apply to any type of inversion:

» The flyer sets up their **upper body foundation**, lifts one leg in the air, and waits for the spotter to get into position.

» The **spotter supports the lifted ankle of the flyer** with the foot resting on their shoulder. (*Spotters: make sure to stand to the outside of the flyer's leg so you don't get kicked accidentally!*)

» Once the spotter is in place, the **flyer slowly pushes their supported foot down** to lift their other leg up.

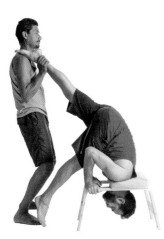 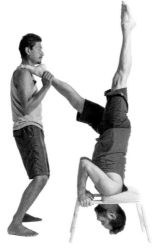 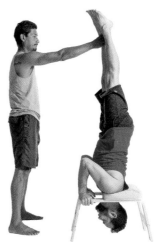

Spotter Supports One Leg   Flyer "Scissor-Lifts" Free Leg   Spotter Extends Arm

» The **spotter can extend their arm** when the flyer's free leg is vertical.

» Finally once the flyer is stable, the spotter needs to move out of the way or go to the flyer's back side.

Hot Potato

This spotting technique is straight out of your childhood backyard! In Hot Potato the spotter supports the flyer by offering **frequent, light assists that allow the flyer to feel their own weight** and find their own balance. This is important because as a spotter, if you never let go, the flyer will develop a dependency and will not learn to balance without support.

Spotters should be near the hips or thighs of the flyer to support leg alignment during the inversion, and be ready to move to Hands On Spotting at the hips for the exit.

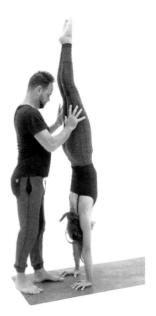

Hot Potato Spotting

Safety Spot

When a flyer is ready to attempt a skill without a spotter for the first time, a Safety Spot is a great way to give some freedom and support. The spotter stands at the side with **one or both arms extended at chest height**, parallel to the ground. You are more or less **like an interactive wall giving space** for the flyer to feel free, but **jumping in to block** them if they go beyond vertical.

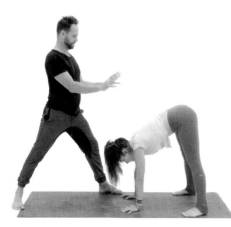

Safety Spotter in Position

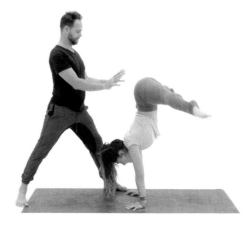

Spotter's Hands Ready

SOLO INVERSIONS TO PRACTICE

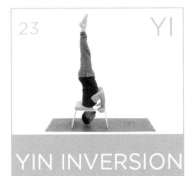

Yin Inversion (YI)

FOUNDATION: Shoulders resting on the seats of two chairs, head between chairs, hands holding chair legs.

ACTIONS: Invert whole body until vertical; breathe mindfully and relax shoulders.

SPOTTING: Behind the flyer, Hands On for beginners.

BENEFITS: Safe way for beginners to invert; massages the shoulders and upper body.

PROPS NEEDED: Two stable chairs against a wall. Make sure they are wide enough apart to fit your head comfortably between them. You can place folded towels under each shoulder for more padding if desired.

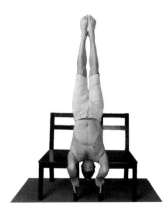

Yin Inversion on Chairs

» Place your **head between the chairs**, hands holding the chair legs, fingers pointed down.

» Scissor-Lift entry is ideal if you have a spotter. If not, either **Tuck (Tu) jump or lift one leg** and swing it up to get your hips over your head. As you are inverting, **push toward the floor** to make your ascent more successful.

» Once inverted, you can use the support of the wall as much or as little as needed. **Practice Range of Motion (ROM)** pressing in Tuck (Tu), Straddle (Str), and Pike (Pi).

» Be sure to **breathe and relax** your shoulders while inverted.

» *Do a child's pose after you come down for 3–5 breaths.*

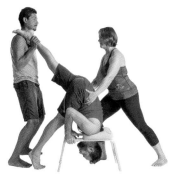

Scissor-Lift and Hands On Spotting for Yin Inversion

Shoulderstand (Sh)

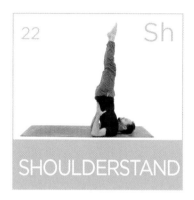

FOUNDATION: Head, neck, shoulders, and triceps; elbows beneath hands, hands supporting the back.

ACTIONS: Invert lower body until vertical, lifting legs overhead; listen to neck health and adjust, breathing mindfully.

BENEFITS: Offers a platform to do many inverted leg variations without the fear of falling.

CHALLENGES: Neck and upper back restriction or pain.

Practice: Tuck Up to Shoulderstand

» Lie down on your back with your arms by your side, palms facing the floor.

» While pushing your arms into the floor, tuck your knees into your chest.

» Once your hips rise up enough you can place your palms under your hips or lower back.

» From this platform created by your arms, you can see your legs and practice Range of Motion (ROM) drills. *See next page.*

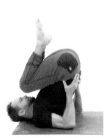 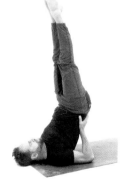 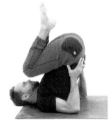

Tuck Up and Support Hips   Extend to Shoulderstand   Return to Tuck

Tuck (Tu): In tuck you bend at the hips and knees, bringing your feet as close to your butt as possible. This leg position is useful for flyers who don't have enough hamstring flexibility to keep their legs straight as they move them.

Practice: Leg Position Range of Motion (ROM)

For each of these variations, start in a Straight Shoulderstand (Sh), move into the leg position, then return to Straight.

Pike (Pi): Pike is the equivalent of folding at the hips. In this variation, the flyer's legs are together as they bring their thighs closer to their belly.

Practicing Pike helps you find unification because you learn to squeeze your legs together as you move them.

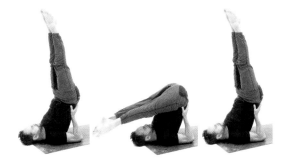

PIKE

Open Straddle (OStr): Here the flyer's legs only move in one direction: apart from each other, without any pike.

This leg variation is very useful because it allows a base to see their flyer's feet without affecting the flyer's straightness.

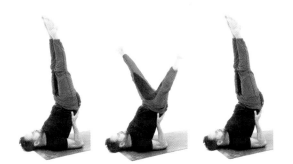

STRADDLE

Piked Straddle (PiStr): Here the legs move in two directions: apart from each other *and* toward the belly.

Piked Straddle is essential for many L-Base skills where the tops of the flyer's thighs create the platform for the base's feet to support them.

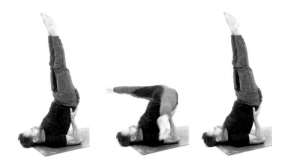

PIKED STRADDLE

Headstand (hs)

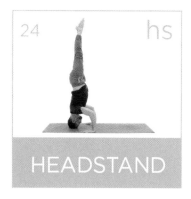

24   hs

HEADSTAND

FOUNDATION: Top of the head, palms on the floor with elbows directly over hands.

ACTIONS: Push down into the hands; keep the body aligned and the neck pain-free; breathe mindfully.

SPOTTING: Behind the flyer, Hands On for beginners.

BENEFITS: Teaches how to invert; is a foundational skill in the jourey to learning handstand.

CHALLENGES: Neck pain.

There are two variations of headstand; the difference is in the foundation. The first, called *Sirsasana A*, utilizes the support of your forearms on the floor with elbows approximately shoulder width apart. The benefit to this variation is that you can protect your neck by pushing your forearms into the floor, taking weight off the head.

The second variation, called *Sirsasana B* or Tripod Headstand, utilizes the palms on the floor with forearms stacked vertically. This variation is more versatile and helps you understand how to push into your palms with vertical forearms; as a flyer you will use this same technique in inverted partner poses and many flying transitions.

Once you've set up your foundation, the rest of the exercise on the following page is the same for both variations.

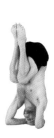

Tuck Up to
Headstand

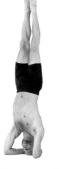

Sirsasana A

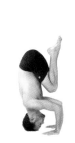

Tuck Up to
Tripod Headstand

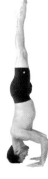

Sirsasana B

Practice: Headstand Against a Wall

First, a Note on Headstands:

With enthusiasm for their benefits, many yoga teachers choose to share headstands with beginner students. While I agree there is much to gain from them, the practice of headstands involves a very real potential for neck injuries.

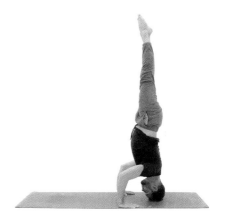

I do not recommend attempting headstands until you are very comfortable with Shoulderstand (Sh) and have done many Yin Inversions (YI) on chairs. In my experience, headstands can one of the most challenging inversions to do safely.

Everyone's necks and skulls are unique, but correct alignment in a headstand should generally feel the same for all. You want to have your head in a neutral position (not angled forward or flexed back), and find a stable, comfortable place where you can breathe.

When you feel ready to attempt a headstand, follow these instructions:

» **Set up your foundation** against a wall.

» Either **Tuck (Tu) jump or lift one leg** and swing it up to get your hips over your head.

» As you are inverting, **push toward the floor** to make your ascent more successful.

» Once inverted, you can **use the wall's support** as much as you need. Practice pressing in Tuck (Tu), Straddle (Str), and Pike (Pi) Range of Motion (ROM).

» **Be sure to breathe** while inverted.

» *Do a child's pose after you come down for 3–5 breaths.*

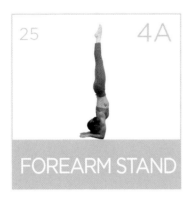

Forearm Stand (4A)

FOUNDATION: Forearms on floor, fingers interlaced or flat on the floor, elbows under shoulders.

ACTIONS: Push into the floor; unify the body.

SPOTTING: Scissor-Lift then transition to the back. Hands On at the hips to come down. Safety Spot from the side for intermediate students learning how to move away from needing a spotter.

BENEFITS: Opens, strengthens, and aligns the shoulders.

CHALLENGES: Shoulder tightness.

Practice: Scissor-Lift to Forearm Stand ATB (Alignment, Tightness, Balance)

Step One:
SCISSOR-LIFT

» Place **palms together, hands interlaced** (or flat on the floor with arms parallel) and head neutral.

» **Have your spotter Scissor-Lift** you into the forearm stand. *(See page 223 for Scissor-Lift.)*

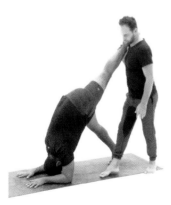
Forearm Stand Prep

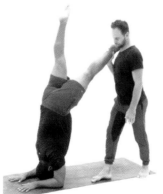
Scissor-Lift

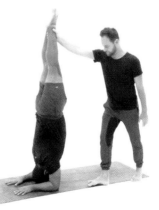
Flyer Inverts, Feet Together

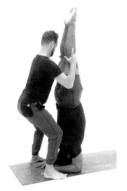

Spotter Lifts to Align

Step Two:
ALIGNMENT

» Once stable, keep your head neutral and wait for your spotter to walk around to your back. The spotter **lifts the flyer up from their thighs** to align the forearm stand as tall and as straight as the flyer's flexibility allows.

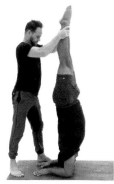

Spotter Tests Leg Tightness

Step Three:
TIGHTNESS

» Next the spotter tries to **pull the flyer's legs apart** as the flyer holds them together. This is meant to **activate the flyer's leg muscles** and their willpower to engage them.

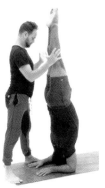

Flyer Looks Down to Balance

Step Four:
BALANCE

» Finally, the flyer slowly lifts their gaze in between their thumbs as the spotter goes to a **Hot Potato spotting** technique, doing the minimum. Be sure to breathe while inverted.

» To come down the spotter returns to Hands On spotting at the hips.

» *Do a child's pose after you come down for 3–5 breaths.*

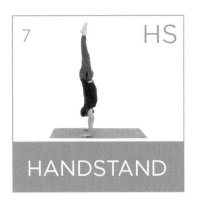

Handstand (HS)

FOUNDATION: Hands shoulder width apart, fingers spread wide, middle fingers parallel.

ACTIONS: Push down into the floor.

SECONDARY ACTIONS: Unify the body by engaging all the muscles; breathe mindfully.

BENEFITS: Unlocks gymnastics and partner acrobatics skills.

CHALLENGES: Arm injuries or lack of mobility in the arms; difficulty making the body straight or balancing; not knowing how to come down safely.

Practice: Scissor-Lift to Handstand ATB (Alignment, Tightness, Balance)

Step One:
SCISSOR-LIFT

» Begin with fingers spread as wide as possible, middle fingers parallel to each other, **hands under the shoulders**, elbows straight, and head neutral.

» **Have your spotter Scissor-Lift** you into the handstand. (*See page 223 for Scissor-Lift.*)

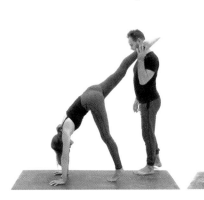
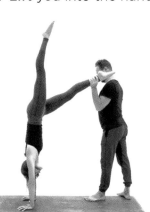
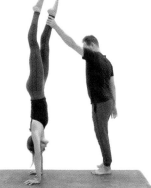

| Handstand Prep | Scissor-Lift | Flyer Inverts, Feet Together |

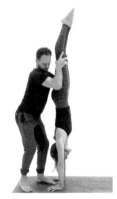

Spotter Lifts to Align

Step Two:
ALIGNMENT

» Once stable, keep your head neutral and wait for your spotter to walk around to your back. The spotter **lifts the flyer up from their thighs** to align the handstand as tall and as straight as the flyer's flexibility allows.

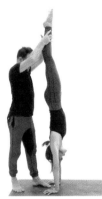

Spotter Tests Leg Tightness

Step Three:
TIGHTNESS

» Next the spotter tries to **pull the flyer's legs apart** as the flyer holds them together. This is meant to **activate the flyer's leg muscles** and their willpower to engage them.

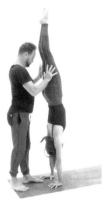

Flyer Looks Down to Balance

Step Four:
BALANCE

» Finally, the flyer slowly lifts their gaze in between their thumbs as the spotter goes to a **Hot Potato spotting** technique, doing the minimum. Be sure to breathe while inverted.

» To come down the spotter returns to Hands On spotting at the hips.

» *Do a child's pose after you come down for 3–5 breaths.*

PARTNER INVERSIONS TO PRACTICE

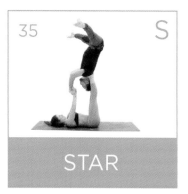

Star (S)

FOUNDATION: Hand to Hand Grip, highest part of the flyer's shoulders resting in the lowest part of the arch of the base's feet. Once stable, the base can lock their heels together to give the flyer a new contact point between their head and the base's shins.

BASE ACTIONS: With knees bent and arms straight or half bent and stable, wait until flyer is over your feet, then extend legs vertically. Hands and arms offer more support in the beginning and can become more and more free as the partners get more calibrated.

FLYER ACTIONS: Stand at the base's head, lower your shoulders to their feet, jump and press into the inversion.

SPOTTING: Behind the base's legs, spine straight.

BENEFITS: This is the downward dog of flying transitions—there are many flying flows that go through Star; best way to enter into Hand to Hand for new bases and flyers; can relax and release the shoulders and trapezius muscles.

CHALLENGES: The base needs to be patient, waiting to extend their legs until the flyer gets their center of gravity over the base; non-optimal foot placement can cause skin burn or injure the flyer's upper body.

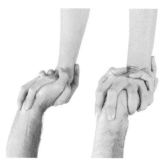

Hand to Hand Grip

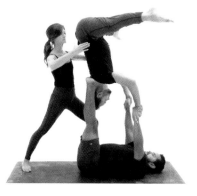

Spotting for Star: At the Back, Hands On the Hips

Practice: Progression to Star (S)

Step One:
SET YOUR FOUNDATION—*PREP WITH PILLOW STAR*

» The base sits with their **legs straight, heels touching**, and feet open.

» Flyer lays on their back and **gently places their head** on the base's shins.

» They take a **Hand to Hand Grip**, flyer with bent arms to line their forearms up with the base's straight arms.

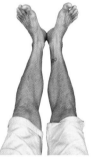
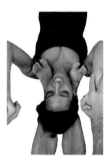
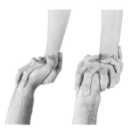

Base's Feet Alignment   Pillow Star   Hand to Hand Grip

Step Two:
SPOTTING AND FLYER ACTION—*PREP WITH HANDS-ON JUMP TO PIKED STRADDLE HANDSTAND*

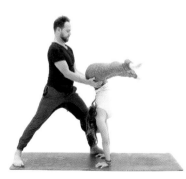

Jump to Piked Straddle
Handstand

» Flyer sets up in a **Chihuahua Dog (CD)**, spotter in a Warrior 1 (W1) pose with their front foot outside the flyer's pinky finger.

» **Spotter offers Hands On spotting** by placing their hands at the flyer's hips.

» Flyer **jumps to a Piked Straddle (PiStr) Handstand (HS)**, as spotter gives the support needed to get the flyer inverted.

Step Three:
BASE ACTION—*PREP WITH THRONE PRESSES*

This prep is designed to help the base learn how to do two critical things: bend their arms and legs effectively, and stack their arms and legs vertically.

When a flyer tries to jump into Star (S), the more the base can bend their legs, the less height the flyer will need in their jump to get over the base's feet. This is why base Range of Motion (ROM) is very advantageous in Star.

Next, if a base is able to stack the bones of their arms and legs vertically, they need less muscle to hold the flyer up. *(See Bones Are Stronger than Muscles page 24.)* This drill familiarizes the base with the distinction between bent versus straight. It also activates the muscles a base will need not just to help the flyer get inverted, but also to support them with stability once in the pose.

> » From Throne (T) *(see page 169)* the **base bends their arms and legs evenly and equally, then extends both**. This Range of Motion is what they will need to support the flyer inverting to Star (S) on their feet.

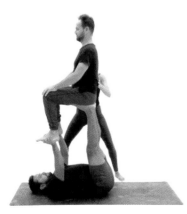 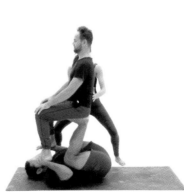 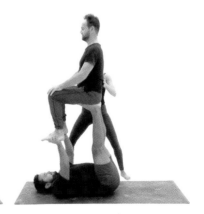

| Begin in Throne | Base Range of Motion: Bend Arms & Legs | Return to Throne |

Step Four:
JUMP TO STAR (S)

» Flyer stands with their **feet at the base's shoulders**. Base presents arms extended and vertical.

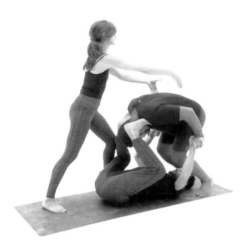

Jump to Star Prep

» Base and flyer take a **Hand to Hand Grip** and flyer bends their arms and pushes into the base to feel their support.

» **Flyer lowers their shoulders** onto the base's feet.

» Spotter stands at the flyer's back with **Hands On the flyer's hips**.

» Flyer **jumps up into the inversion** as the spotter supports. The base keeps their legs bent and arms straight and stable.

» Once the flyer is fully inverted and over the base's feet, the base can **extend their legs to vertical**.

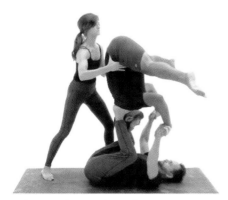

Spotter is Hands on for Jump Entry

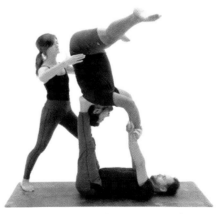

Once Inverted, Base Extends

Step Five:
STAR (S) RANGE OF MOTION (ROM) PRESSES

This individual and joint Range of Motion (ROM) training will help you enter Star (S) with more ease, and progress to using Star (S) in flying transitions.

» Once in a stable Star, the **base stays still and stable as the flyer experiments** with Tuck (Tu), Pike (Pi), and Straddle (Str) Range of Motion (ROM) presses. *See page 240 for Leg Positions.*

» Then the **flyer stays still and stable as the base explores** their Range of Motion (ROM) with squats and rotating their flyer from side to side by swiveling their legs.

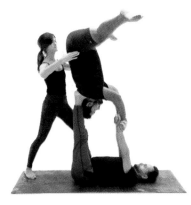
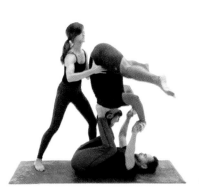
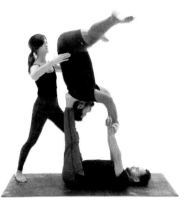

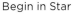

| Begin in Star | Base Bends Legs | Base Straightens Legs |

» Once each partner is individually calibrated, **try jointly exploring your Range of Motion (ROM)**. The base bends their legs as the flyer presses down in a Piked Straddle (PiStr), and then extends their legs as the flyer simultaneously presses back to vertical.

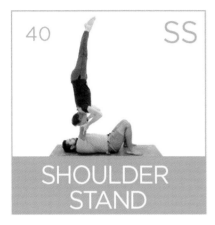

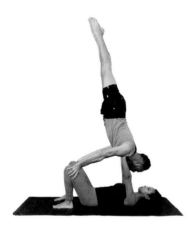

Supported Shoulderstand,
aka "Candlestick"

Shoulder Stand (SS)

FOUNDATION: Highest part of the flyer's shoulder on the lowest part of the base's palm, base's thumbs in line with other fingers; flyer's palms resting on the base's forearms with their fingers pointing toward the floor.

BASE ACTIONS: Receive the flyer's weight and keep arms straight.

FLYER ACTIONS: Lower your shoulders into the base's hands and invert over the base's arms, elbows in; look down, and push down into the base's support.

SPOTTING: From the back, hands near hips.

BENEFITS: Many variations possible and, like Star (S), is in many flying transitions; many variations possible in grip, hand placement, and contact points for both base and flyer—each with its own advantages and limitations.

CHALLENGES: Base's wrists can be compressed if alignment is off; can be hard for the base to support the flyer if they fall toward their back.

DRILLS: Candlestick Shoulderstand with Tuck (Tu), Pike (Pi), and Straddle (Str) presses. *(See following page.)*

Practice: Candlestick Shoulderstand

» **Base lies down on their back** with their feet as close to their butt as possible. The flyer steps over the base's knees in a Straddle (Str).

» Base reaches toward the flyer's shoulders with straight arms as the **flyer lowers their upper body** toward the base. The flyer's hands hold the base's knees.

» **Spotter stands at the back** in a Warrior 1 (W1) Stance *(see page 152)* with Hands On the flyer's hips.

» Then the flyer can **climb to the knees of the base** in a Tuck (Tu) and **press up from there** to the Candlestick Shoulderstand.

» Once inverted and stable, the flyer can do Tuck (Tu), Pike (Pi), and Straddle (Str) Range of Motion (ROM) presses. Spotter is Hands On but doing as little as possible.

PREP

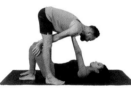

Candlestick Shoulderstand Prep

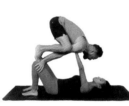

Flyer Climbs to Base's Knees

TUCK

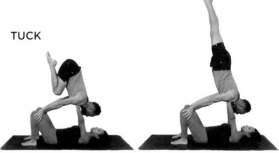

Tuck (Tu) Press

Candlestick Shoulderstand

PIKE

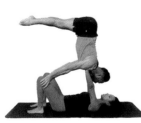

Pike (Pi) Press

Candlestick Shoulderstand

STRADDLE

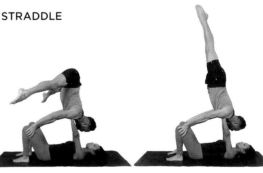

Straddle (Str) Press

Candlestick Shoulderstand

PART V
HEALING IS OUR BIRTHRIGHT

Healing is as natural as getting hurt; we do both every day to some degree. Yet in modern society we often give our power to medical professionals, forgetting that we all have access to natural healing and nurturing practices. It's our birthright to reclaim access to our body's inherent healing systems.

No other animal on earth goes to hospitals; billions of happy, healthy creatures out there are doing many things right to have the health that they do. Being healthy is the norm when we are aligned with our nature and the life force within us.

In this section you will learn how to fill your body with vitality through breath control, and how to move that energy through your body with mindfulness practices. You will also learn one of the most powerful ways to make friends and help people giggle: therapeutic flying! This is how I become instant friends with anyone who says yes to the question, "Wanna fly?"

15

EVERYTHING CAN BE A MEDITATION

When the breath is unsteady, all is unsteady; when the breath is still; all is still. Control the breath carefully. Inhalation gives strength and a controlled body; retention gives steadiness of mind and longevity; exhalation purifies body and spirit.
—GORAKSHA SATAKAM

Your breath is your first gift. You have a limited number of breaths to enjoy in this life. Your first breath may be your most enthusiastic one; your last one may be your softest. The quality of each breath will influence the quality of your mind, your emotions, and in turn, your life. You can train your mind and breath with various mindfulness practices, or you can live a long life with little attention to these facets of your experience. This chapter is dedicated to the power of mindfulness—the practice of bringing your conscious attention to something fully. By honing your mindfulness skills, everything you do can open you up to deeper levels of awareness and connection.

Breath and meditation are two gateways to mindfulness and are easy, powerful actions you can take to support all aspects of your well-being. Imagine your entire body as a glass of muddy water. The glass is your skin, the water is your true self, and the mud is all the chaos, negativity, and suffering inside you. Just by sitting still and "meditating," the mud will naturally settle to the bottom of the glass. Focusing on your breath is like attaching a little pool filter to your glass that will pull the chaos and negativity out of your system.

Nobody can breathe or meditate for you; this is your work alone, and doing it will prime you to show up for others in a centered and authentic way. The more partner work you do, the more vital these personal practices are for you to distill who you are when the chaos settles. The sections to follow draw on the wisdom from my own practices and studies to guide you through incorporating breathwork and meditation into your life. By trying these tools you will be able to determine for yourself how you can bring your best self forward.

HOW TO GET MORE OUT OF EACH BREATH

Keep a close watch on the breath: outside and inside, stopped or being exchanged. Observe too, the place in the body, the duration, and the count, long and subtle.
—*YOGA SUTRAS OF PATAÑJALI,* 2.50
TRANSLATED BY GESHE MICHAEL ROACH

There is an entire branch of yoga practices dedicated to breath called *pranayama,* Sanskrit for "breath control." *Prana* means "life force"—on a subtle level, it's what is vibrating in our atoms, the neurotransmitters facilitating our consciousness, our breath, our thoughts, and our blood. Anything that moves is related to your *prana. Yama* means "control." We have all controlled our breath as we've blown out birthday candles, swam underwater, or blown up a balloon. We cannot escape breath because if we do it's game over for us. With too much oxygen, we risk becoming dizzy, experiencing seizures and losing consciousness. With too little oxygen, we die. But between those extremes, there is a lot of room to play with directing energy through our bodies by controlling the breath. Breath is a miniature life cycle: the inhale is being born; the exhale is dying. Inhalation is about the feeding and filling of your inner world; exhalation is about surrender and softening to your external world. None of us are getting out of here alive, so we may as well allow the breath to teach us as much as it can about gathering energy and letting it go.

Take the time to practice your awareness of when you are moving your breath and stopping it. You can breathe space, vitality, and energy to different places in your body as you gain mastery of this limb of yoga. Monitoring the duration by counting your breath is an easy way to keep your mind busy with something simple. This can be your gateway to a meditative state. Breaths can be long and subtle as your practice grows, and this type of breathing will bring the many parts of you into alignment. You have to establish a practice and do the experiments to get better at *pranayama*.

Pranayama is a very rhythmic and scientific practice with different techniques to either give the body more energy or calm it down. In a greater sense, breath control translates to mental, physical, and emotional control. One way to measure it is by how long you can hold breath in your body, and how long you can hold it outside of your body. You can also measure it by how effectively you can shift your mood. For example, if I am able to take a deep breath before I respond to my partner or before I engage in a tense moment, chances are I will have more success with a harmonious exchange of information. A regular practice of three to five minutes of breathing to start or finish your meditation or yoga practice is a great way to incorporate the gifts of breathwork.

In yoga, breath is everything. The rhythm of your inhalations and exhalations synchronizes all your movements in the practice. The inhale helps the body to lengthen, open, and expand into a pose. The exhale allows a softening or release, settling into the bones and the earth. The inhale draws

prana in and up through the body; the exhale grounds the body, sending energy down as tension and toxins are released.

In solar AcroYoga practices, the inhale is used to sync up the timing of dynamic actions. It is a way to see, hear, and feel two different bodies starting to move as one. The exhale is when force is applied: the muscles fire up and the dynamic skill is brought into motion. The more advanced your AcroYoga practice becomes, the more you and your partner's breath become connected. This becomes one of the markers of advancement in your partnerships.

In lunar therapeutic practices, givers attend and respond to the breath of the receiver, and the two may sync their breaths as well. The inhale allows the giver to draw in potential energy, adjust points of contact, and prepare to apply pressure. The exhale is when pressure, a twist, a bend, or traction is applied. For the receiver, the inhale collects *prana* or potential healing energy and creates a bit of tension throughout the whole body from the pressure in the lungs and chest. On the exhale, the body softens to receive the action of the giver. Moving with breath awareness is already a powerful, embodied meditation practice. Next I will present more ideas for you to go deeper into the subtle world of meditation.

MEDITATION

In my teenage years I worked at a fish store. I learned how to say the name of the state fish of Hawaii, *Humuhumunukunukuapua'a,* meaning "the triggerfish with a snout like a pig." I also learned how to care for sick fish. Whenever we got new fish in, we would put them in their own tank for a few days. If they showed signs of weakness it was usually because they had parasites. To address this we would introduce them to a harsh but healing environment. The freshwater fish would go into a saltwater tank and the saltwater fish would go into a freshwater tank. The idea is that in a harsh environment the weaker parasite will die and the stronger organism will live. Until the treatment, the invaders were drawing the fish's attention and life force. It was only successful if the treatment lasted for the right duration of time. Not enough time and the parasite lived on; too much time and the fish itself would be endangered. Why this story of fish, you ask?

During my meditation practice this kind of cleansing is exactly what I go through most mornings. The parasites change from day to day: fear of not making enough money, desire to look at my phone to see what is happening on my Instagram page, scattered agitated thinking, etc. If you have time to brush your teeth and check your phone, you have time to meditate. You can do it while you wait at the DMV or while you wait for your partner to come watch a movie with you; there is always time in the day to take some mindful moments and slow down. I have experienced, like in all practices, that the more I dedicate the more benefit I receive, but also that I have to get hooked by the little investments.

By design, the mind is a busy bee. As much as the mind can train the body, in moments of stillness and focus the body can also train the mind. Taking time to trap this busy bee in a calm, seated meditation can kill the many potential parasites of the mind which would otherwise eat away at your mental peace. Your friends, lovers, colleagues, and AcroYoga partners can help and support you in your struggles, but they cannot do your work for you. Meditation is you doing your own self-love practice. The more you discover in your own meditation practice, the better you will be at sharing your life with others.

To complement the sometimes wild, high-energy qualities of AcroYoga is the act of slowing everything down and listening to your individual body. The word "meditation" comes from the Latin *meditari,* meaning "to meditate, think over, reflect, consider." Meditation does not have to be seated with your eyes closed. It also happens in the midst of movement, while completing mundane activities, or in moments of profound connection with others.

Indeed, everything can be a meditation. When the body and mind are in their lanes the bumps that life offers are much less jarring. The mind being centered and focused lets the body know that everything is okay. What is more important than how or why you meditate is simply dedicating time to doing the practice so that you can become meditative.

RAJA YOGA FOR ACROYOGIS

Raja yoga brings the mind, body, and breath into alignment. *Raja* means "king",

and this practice is considered one of the jewels of yoga. Many of these practices start with a steady, comfortable seated pose. You want to be comfortable so you can stay long enough to receive the benefits. Sit on something so your knees are at or below the height of your hips. Find a tall spine, close your eyes, and breathe.

How long is long enough? Start small and listen. A few minutes is a great way to start or end your day. Once you do seven days in a row of meditation you will see what the benefits are for you. Often in the beginning meditation is a way to calm down an overactive mind. Over time you might gain clarity in areas of your life where you have conflict, or even come up with your next life calling. The amazing thing about meditation is you don't need anything to do it. Just like handstands, however, you actually have to *do* it to improve at it.

In the *Yoga Sūtras* there are three progressive steps that lead practitioners to a meditative state of consciousness:

1. PRATYAHARA: withdrawal from the senses
2. DHĀRAṆA: concentration
3. DHYĀNA: meditation

Each of these three stages offers lessons and benefits for practitioners of AcroYoga.

STEP 1: PRATYAHARA— WITHDRAWAL FROM THE SENSES

If you close your eyes, your sense of hearing improves. If you plug your ears, you can feel your heartbeat more easily. The more we limit our sensory perception the more finely we can tune our whole body as an instrument of awareness.

Our senses can be thought of as many horses drawing a carriage (your body) steered by a driver (your mind). The horses are often stampeding, pulling the carriage in different directions, and the driver, from time to time, loses hold of the reins. *Pratyahara* is like the driver grabbing hold of the reins and bringing the stampeding horses to a halt. Now she can inspect the carriage, look around at where they are, and consult her map. When we withdraw from the senses, we gain profound insight into ourselves and how we relate to our environment, without distraction or confusion.

Sensory withdrawal sharpens our perceptions as it forces us to become more sensitive: if you close your eyes and walk across the room, you feel the texture of the floor and hear the sound of your feet with a new level of attention. AcroYoga can at times be a very big, in-your-face kind of practice. *Pratyahara* helps us to balance high sensory intake and digest everything we're learning during training.

There are many ways to apply this to your AcroYoga practice. You can take a round of flying where the base is the one speaking and the flyer just listens. After one round you switch. You can do Thai massage blindfolded to learn to see with your hands more clearly. As you take senses away your awareness sharpens.

STEP 2: DHĀRAṆA— CONCENTRATION

Acrobats spend countless hours in a state of high-stakes concentration. If a yogi blinks during a candle-gazing practice, there is no risk of injury; but if I lose focus while throwing my partner in the air, there are huge risks for both of us. For this reason, I believe acrobats and AcroYogis already have a huge capacity to understand the practice of *Dhāraṇa*.

Concentration is a gateway into the present moment. The modern world is rife with distractions that pull our focus into the past, future, and alternative made-up worlds. But we were made to live in the present. Our ancestors had to spend much of their lives concentrating on the tasks before them, remaining alert to constantly emerging dangers and opportunities: predators, prey, water sources, weather patterns, etc. Risk, joy, competition, and celebration are just some of the ways we are invited to move naturally from scattered attention to *Dhāraṇa*—using our senses with maximum focus. *Dhāraṇa* is the opposite of multitasking; it is a mental multivitamin that prepares the mind for meditation.

STEP 3: DHYĀNA— MEDITATION

Dhyāna is the training of the mind to unhook itself from automatic reactions to sensory information, thereby leading to a "state of perfect equanimity and awareness." This means that while the horses may still be pushing and pulling in seven different directions, the driver has such a confident, firm grip on the reins that the carriage is not pulled off course. I might have just snorted a lump of high-grade wasabi up one nostril, but in a state of *Dhyāna*, no amount of sensory overload would break my equanimity. This equally applies to positive stimulation, which can also wreak havoc on our peace of mind. Think of how distracted we become by candy or toys as children, or by the excitement of a new romantic interest once we get a little older. Whether the horses are driven by fear or tempted by a carrot, if they overwhelm the driver and crash the carriage, the result is the same.

In AcroYoga it can be easy to feel frustrated when we don't nail a new skill, but it can also be easy to get so excited about a success that we become lazy or unfocused in subsequent attempts. In either headspace people can easily get hurt. Remembering *Dhyāna*—calm, non-reaction to positive or negative stimuli—can help us rein the horses back in when they risk getting out of control. You can apply these ancient seeds of widsom to your life in the time-tested principles that follow.

MEDITATION PRINCIPLES

1. Be Consistent.

You might be thinking, *Are you for real? Not again!* Yes, I am for real, and here it is again! To practice mindfulness, you have to bring your attention, focus, and love into what you do with consistency.

Meditation can become a large part of your life. In fact, some saints and sages are presumably in meditation most of the day. It could be a seated meditation for three minutes per day before you sleep or when you wake. It could be taking five deep breaths before turning your phone on.

Where you apply the practices is less important than having a consistent practice and digging deep enough to find the benefits.

2. Inhale, Exhale, Repeat.

There is no better singular activity you can do to reduce all the chaos of life into the present moment than breathing. We can push the reset button on so many of our systems with the simple, essential act of deeply filling and fully emptying our lungs.

The quality of your breath and the quality of your life are tied together. Get good at breathing and you will get better at life.

3. Being Present Is a Gift.

Meditation is not just done by sitting on a cushion with your eyes closed. It can be felt and practiced in all aspects of your life. When you are engaged and excited by what you are doing, this is a doorway to meditation.

The word "present" itself clearly says that every moment is a gift! Any and all real things happen in the state of being present. It is a place where fear of the future cannot exist and sadness of the past cannot haunt us.

We are at our best on many levels when we are present. We can focus all of our talent and resources on what we are doing. We can avoid getting lost in the myriad of theories about ourselves, others, or the world at large.

It is not that the past and future do not have value; being aware of them can certainly guide us in the direction we want to go. But as we are increasingly present with where we are, we can actualize these precious steps toward our goals more mindfully and efficiently.

Simply by doing AcroYoga you will be invited into the present moment. This is the subtle, unspoken gift of doing this practice.

BREATHING PRACTICES

Three-Part Breathing

This is often the first breathing technique taught to new yoga practitioners. The three parts are the abdomen, diaphragm, and chest. During three-part breathing, you completely fill yourself with air as though you are breathing into your belly first, rib cage second, and upper chest third. Then you exhale completely, reversing the flow from top to bottom. Pick an amount of time between three to five minutes and fill yourself with this caffeine-free buzz of energy.

Ujjayi

The Sanskrit word *Ujjayi* means "to conquer or be victorious." *Ujjayi Pranayama* is one breathing technique that helps calm the mind and warm the body. When practicing *Ujjayi*, you completely fill your lungs by breathing through your nose while slightly contracting your throat, so your breath becomes audible. This breathing technique is used throughout many different styles of *hatha yoga* practices due to its ability to warm the body from the inside.

Kapalabhati aka "Skull-Polishing Breath"

The word *kapal* means "skull" and *bhati* means "shining or illuminating." *Kapalabhati Pranayama* earned this name because it is said to cleanse or polish the airways inside the head.

   Kapalabhati involves forcefully pulling your navel toward your spine as you expel the breath out through the nose. The exhalation is active and the inhalation is passive. This creates a very slight carbon dioxide debt in your body, so that when you move on to practice slower-paced breathing, your breath is longer and deeper, and it's easier to enter a calm and meditative state. *Kapalabhati* is a very powerful breathing technique that is not recommended for those with heart conditions or high or low blood pressure.

MEDITATION PRACTICES

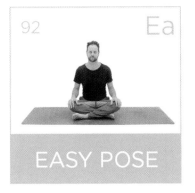

92   Ea

EASY POSE

Seated Meditation

This is the most common type of meditation. In the AcroYoga Table of Elements there are many different seated positions in which you can practice meditation.

Here are six keys to getting the most out of your seated meditation practice:

» You need to find a **comfortable way to sit**. This could be on the floor, on cushions, or in a chair depending on the flexibility of your hips. No matter the position, you want your **knees to be at or below the height of your hips**, and not higher.

» Your **spine should be as straight** as possible.

» Create an **intention or visualization**: *I will be focused, I will be peaceful, I will cultivate acceptance, I will pray for my mom,* etc.

» Do any of the **breathing exercises** listed on the previous page, or any other you know, to bring yourself into a state of focus.

» **Then relax the breath** and allow yourself to witness your thoughts, staying still in your body and steady in your breathing.

» **Journaling or reading** inspirational books before or after your meditation can help you get the most out of these sessions.

Walking Meditation

It's all there in the title! The key is to do it super-duper slowly. Walking meditation is the practice of walking with no aim of getting to a physical place; rather, it is walking to feel the very steady, controlled physical movements of your body. It's most powerful to do this in nature and not around a lot of people. If you do it in the busy streets of NYC you are trying a very advanced variation.

Listening Meditation

Ring a bell and try to listen until you hear no more vibration. The act of deep listening is a form of focus that leads to meditation. Ideally the bell, gong, or sound-making device should have a relatively long cycle of sound (10–30 seconds minimum) so you can ring it five to ten times during your practice.

Seeing Meditation—*Trataka*

Trataka is a yogic exercise to help you focus your eyes. Light a candle and watch it as long as you can until you blink. It is common that tears form as you gain control of your blinking and blink less. Start by trying it for three minutes, and expand the time as it serves you.

Partner Meditation

For a partner meditation practice you can simply do any of the meditations above with someone else, or you can do a seated back-to-back meditation. The benefits here are accountability and connection. When you sit back-to-back with a partner, often your breaths will become synchronized and your focus stays more in the present moment.

Eye-Gazing Meditation

Find a partner and a comfortable seat. You might need pillows to find your perfect nest, knees touching your partner's knees, hands resting on your partner's knees. It is not uncommon to feel weird at first and in that weirdness laughter often bubbles up. That's not a bad byproduct, and there is more so stay with it!

Start by focusing on their third eye, or the space just in between the eyebrows. It's less intimate and helps to ground you both. When you feel ready, look into either one of your partner's eyes. Once you are locked eye to eye you will be flooded with oxytocin, a feel-good love drug from your endocrine pharmacy. Seeing and being seen are both powerful states of being, and after a while they merge and the perceived separation between you and your partner evaporates.

You can also do this practice in front of a mirror to connect more deeply with yourself.

Screen-Free Saturdays

As stated at the beginning of this section, everything can be meditation. Many of us are guilty of being sucked into the charm, instant gratification, and dopaminergic responses from our smartphones.

In light of this, it can be a huge life upgrade to unplug from your modern technology-driven life one day per week. Spend time in nature or with your loved ones, enjoying simple pleasures you tend to miss when constantly connected to the quick fix of cyberspace.

Giving your full attention and awareness to the present moment is the aim of this section; this screen-free practice is one way to increase the time available for that aim.

VISIT *WWW.ACROYOGA.ORG/MCP* TO DOWNLOAD A FREE WORKBOOK, WATCH TUTORIALS, AND FIND OUR COMPANION VIDEO COURSE TO HELP YOU ACTIVATE THE PRINCIPLES AND PRACTICES DISCUSSED IN THIS CHAPTER.

16

LUNAR ELEMENTS AND PRACTICES

The lunar therapeutic practices are what make AcroYoga different from most other forms of acrobatics. Here we learn to use the skill and power of acrobatics with the wisdom of Thai massage to care for the body service of its alignment, balance, and healing. AcroYoga thus becomes more sustainable as a lifelong practice.

The lunar arts offer you tools to bring more softness, compassion and harmony into your life and all your relationships. Of all the things one can dedicate to, understanding how to heal and care for your body and your friends' bodies will always be one of the most valuable. As you give, you can feel good and foster a deeper connection to the people you work and play with.

Thai massage is a practice of aligning your body and breath with your receiver's, and letting your bodyweight and presence unwind the tension and stress of life. Thai massage is a yoga practice, a meditation, and a healing dance all in one. All styles of dance have their signature steps and ways of moving that set them apart. We all have the ability to dance, but to begin with a certain style we must first learn the basics.

Thes following stances are the most important steps in the sacred dance of Thai Massage. You can think of them like yoga poses you'll get to do on a human mat. Remember, gravity is the therapist. As we learn to realign with her we learn to move with efficiency and ease while resetting the physical patterns of the body and optimizing recovery after acrobatic training.

THAI STANCES

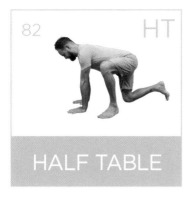

HALF TABLE

Half Table (HT)

FOUNDATION: Foot under knee, other knee under hip, back foot flexed, hands under shoulders.

BENEFITS: Very stable platform to palm your receiver's body.

CHALLENGES: Can be uncomfortable on the back knee if the surface is hard.

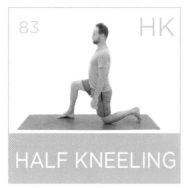

HALF KNEELING

Half Kneeling (HK)

FOUNDATION: Foot under knee, other knee under hip, back foot flexed.

BENEFITS: Very stable; front leg can be used to support receiver's arms and legs; also good for transitioning between stances.

CHALLENGES: Can be uncomfotable on the back knee if the surface is hard.

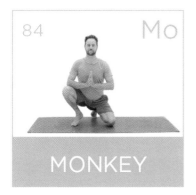

MONKEY

Monkey (Mo)

FOUNDATION: Front foot flat on the ground, back foot flexed with toes spread, back knee supported by the floor.

BENEFITS: When you get low to the ground there are many ways you can use your body to create traction; lots of Thai transitions move in and out of Monkey.

CHALLENGES: Can be intense on the back foot.

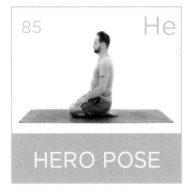

Hero Pose (He)

FOUNDATION: Knees, shins, and tops of the feet.

BENEFITS: Creates a great platform on your thighs to palm, thumb, and roll out your receiver's body; great for performing blood-stops on arms and legs.

CHALLENGES: Can aggravate existing knee or ankle injuries.

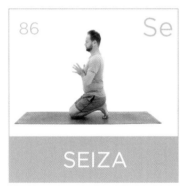

Seiza (Se)

FOUNDATION: Knees and all ten flexed toes.

BENEFITS: Very stable, opens the giver's toes, creates a clear place to pour weight from.

CHALLENGES: Can be intense on the feet.

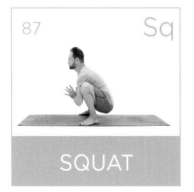

Squat (Sq)

FOUNDATION: Feet flat on the ground with equal weight on all four corners of both feet, or heels up if there is a lack of flexibility.

BENEFITS: This pose is very mobile and grants easy access to a lot of bodyweight; creates space in the lower back, ankle, knee and hip joints.

CHALLENGES: You need a lot of flexibility to be comfortable in this pose; it is not very stable.

RECOVERY AND MEDITATION POSES

One of the byproducts of modern life is that we move fast and often do not get enough rest or have enough ways to release our daily stress. This section is the antidote to an overworked and under-rested body, mind and nervous system.

I chose the following poses for two main purposes: First, they are all great for meditation and solo practices. Second, they translate to self-massage, Thai massage, and shapes for flyers to know before they fly.

If you love the dynamic acrobatic poses, these therapeutic poses can serve as the perfect complement for developing softness, sensitivity and the ability to heal so you can train dynamic acrobatics in a centered way, for many years to come.

Feel free to use a small pillow to make these poses more comfortable.

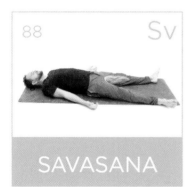

88   Sv

SAVASANA

Savasana (Sv)

FOUNDATION: The entire back of the body.

ACTIONS: Surrender control of breath, muscles, and mind; fully relax from head to toe.

BENEFITS: Integration of practice; integration of body, mind, and spirit; helps to release stress and tension; easiest position for your heart to pump blood to your entire body.

CHALLENGES: A busy mind may keep you from reaching a deeply restful state; can put pressure on the lower back.

VARIATIONS: Bolster or pillow under knees to support lower back.

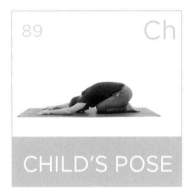

Child's Pose (Ch)

FOUNDATION: Knees, shins, and tops of the feet; hands forward on the floor. Knees can be together or apart; feet can be together or apart.

ACTIONS: Find a comfortable way to relax and breathe.

BENEFITS: Integration of inversions and therapeutic flying; brings relaxation into asana practices and creates passive stretch to increase squat mobility.

CHALLENGES: Knee or ankle injuries or extreme tightness in the legs can limit comfort in this pose.

VARIATIONS: Blanket under the knees; fists in the belly.

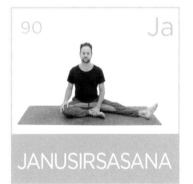

Janusirsasana (Ja)

FOUNDATION: Bottom of the straight leg, outside of the bent leg.

ACTIONS: Sit with a straight spine and breathe into the stretch.

BENEFITS: Opens hamstrings and spine; offers easy access for self-massage on the feet and inner lines of the legs.

CHALLENGES: Hamstring and lower back tightness.

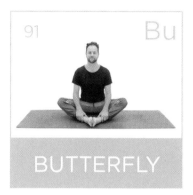

Butterfly (Bu)

FOUNDATION: Sit bones, outer edges of feet and legs, hands at the ankles.

ACTIONS: Move legs up and down like wings; self-massage on feet and legs.

BENEFITS: Teaches flyer's leg positions for therapeutic flying.

CHALLENGES: Hip, lower back, and leg tightness.

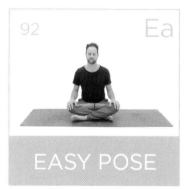

Easy Pose (Ea)

FOUNDATION: Sit bones, outer edges of crossed legs and feet.

ACTIONS: Adjust all the little angles in the feet, legs, and spine to find a stable, comfortable position.

BENEFITS: Ideal for meditation.

CHALLENGES: Hip and lower back tightness.

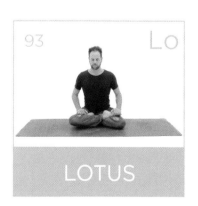

Lotus (Lo)

FOUNDATION: Sit bones and the outer edges of crossed legs with feet on thighs.

ACTIONS: Adjust the angles in the feet, legs, and spine to find a stable, comfortable position.

BENEFITS: Increases blood flow to the upper body as the legs are bound; impresses your friends and strangers alike!

CHALLENGES: Knee and ankle injuries can limit the mobility needed to do this pose.

VARIATIONS: Half lotus; bound lotus.

LUNAR ASANA SEQUENCE

"Vinyasa" is derived from the Sanskrit term nyasa, which means "to place," and the prefix vi, "in a special way"—as in the arrangement of notes in a raga, the steps along a path to the top of a mountain, or the linking of one asana to the next. In the yoga world the most common understanding of vinyasa is a flowing sequence of specific asanas coordinated with the movements of the breath.

—SHIVA REA

This "Vinyasa" yoga sequence brings the lunar elements from the AcroYoga Table of Elements to life. Here, you will take time to practice cultivating your energy by mindfully using your breath in connection with your *yoga asanas*, or physical postures.

The Lunar Asana Sequence is designed to center and heal the body. By doing this sequence you will learn the art of aligning your poses, movement, and breath.

This sequence contains:

1. **Thai stances:** These are the different positions you will need to know to offer Thai massage to your bases after they therapeutically fly you. Think of these stances as the Thai massage alphabet. As you learn how to move in your own body with skill, you will be able to apply that wisdom to how you move in massage.

2. **Qigong:** *Qi* means "energy" and *gong* means "to gather or work." Qigong is an ancient Chinese practice that, on average, is more gentle than yoga and is composed of subtle movements that are typically repeated, or stances that are held, to build and circulate energy.

    At the most subtle level, you are energy. In any mindful movement practice, whether you know it or not, you are connecting to different types of energy and different energy centers in the body. By focusing your mind and breath you can not only connect to the energy in your body, you can learn how to actually control it.

When you know how to move the *prana, qi*, or energy in your body you can more skillfully support your wellness, and whatever you learn to do for yourself can inform how to do that for your friends and partners.

3. **Breath and movement:** One of the first movements in life is the first breath we take when we are born. From our first breath to our last we have a fixed number of breaths to power our actions and align with what we are doing. A key concept in Thai massage is to use the inhalation to set up a foundation and align your body, then use the exhalation to pour your bodyweight. The breath physically moves your body and stretches your tissues, but more importantly, it has the capacity to change your mental and emotional states.

4. **Qualities of touch:** Self-massage plays a big part in the Lunar Asana Sequence. You are your best teacher with touch because you can learn to give the exact amount of pressure that you want. By practicing this sequence, you will get to know your body and learn how to find and release tense muscles.

To follow the sequences on the following pages, move across the pages before starting the next row.

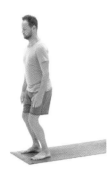
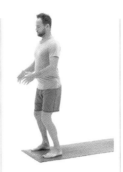
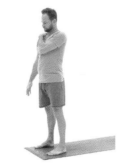
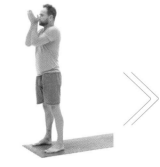

GENERATE & MOVE QI

Stand with feet apart. Bounce and shake limbs freely to stimulate energy in the body, *30–60 sec.*

EARTH PALM

Knees bent, arms rounded, palms down. Feel energy in palms and feet. *3 breaths*

SELF-LOVE HEALING

Place hands on an area of need, *3 breaths*

SELF BLESSING

Inhale hands to face

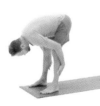
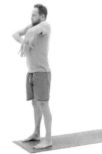
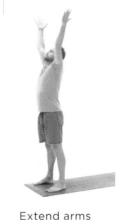
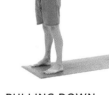

Inhale to draw energy up inner legs

Touch backs of the hands at chest

Extend arms overhead and release energy. *Repeat Self Blessing 3 times*

PULLING DOWN HEAVENS

Begin with arms overhead

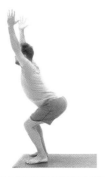
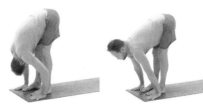
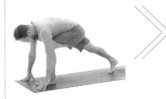

FULL BODY WARM UP

Chair Pose: Feet together, legs bent, arms up, *3 breaths*

UTTANASANA (Ut) FORWARD FOLD & LIFT

Legs straight or bent, exhale relax torso over legs, *3 breaths*. Inhale lift spine halfway, look up

LUNGE

Exhale step right foot back, hands to earth

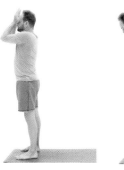
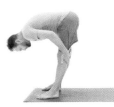
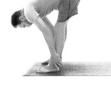

SELF BLESSING

Exhale to softly bathe head and neck with hands

Draw energy down sides of ribs and lower back

Brush down backs of legs

Continue down calves to heels and off the feet

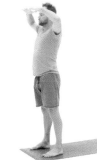
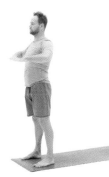
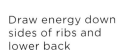
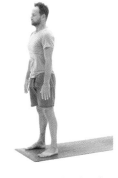
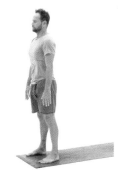

Turn palms to face earth at eye level

Exhale and slowly lower hands, scanning the body

Sense the body. *Repeat Pulling Down Heavens 3 times*

Settle and ground, keeping knees bent, *3 breaths*

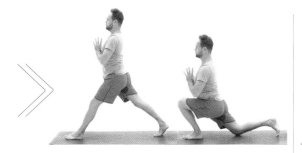
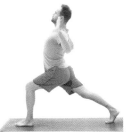
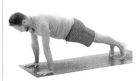

LUNGE PRESS

Inhale raise torso, hands in prayer, back heel lifted. Exhale lower back knee to earth. *Repeat 3 times*

HIGH LUNGE WITH BACK BEND

Inhale to raise back knee, open arms to cactus and Arch (Ar), *3 breaths*

PLANK (PI)

Hands to earth shoulder width apart, arms straight, feet hip width, *3 breaths*

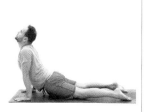

UP DOG

Inhale look up to Arch (Ar), *3 breaths*

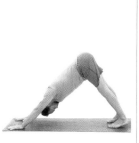

DOWN DOG (DD)

Push hips up and back to Down Dog, *3 breaths*

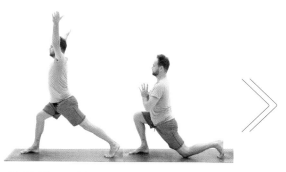

LUNGE PRESS

Step right foot forward, inhale raise torso, arms up, back heel lifted. Exhale lower back knee to earth. *Repeat 3 times*

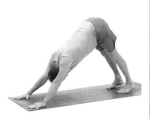

DOWN DOG (DD)

Push hips up and back to open hamstrings, calves, and shoulders, *3 breaths*

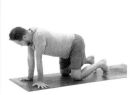

TABLE (TA) PALMING

Lean weight left and right, palming with breath: Inhale to shift weight, exhale to pour weight through straight arms

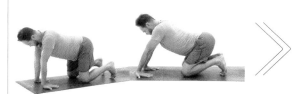

(Ta) WRIST STETCH

Turn hands while palming earth to warm up wrists

Turn fingers to face knees, lean back, *3 breaths*

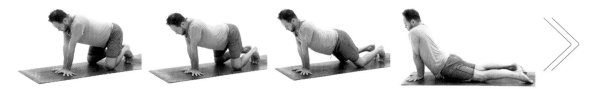

SEIZA (Se) PALMING

Hands to earth, thumbs touching, fingers facing out. Inhale to lean back

Exhale to pour weight through straight vertical arms

Inhale to move hands farther forward, exhale pour weight through straight vertical arms

Inhale to move hands even farther, exhale lower hips to earth, pour weight through straight arms

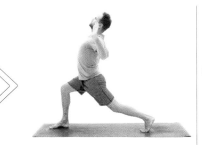

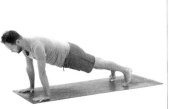

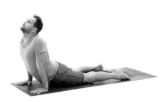

HIGH LUNGE BACK BEND

Inhale raise back knee, open arms to cactus and Arch (Ar), *3 breaths*

PLANK (Pl)

Step back to Plank, arms vertical, *3 breaths*

UP DOG

Inhale Arch (Ar); when aligned the spine and neck will feel good, *3 breaths*

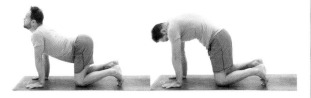

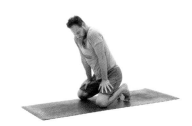

(Ta) SPINE RANGE OF MOTION (ROM)

Inhale look up to Arch (Ar), relax shoulders. Exhale look at belly to Hollow (Ho), extend shoulders. *Repeat 3 times*

SEIZA (Se) PALMING TECHNIQUE

Inhale sit back to Seiza (Se), toes flexed and spread. Palm thighs with fingers facing out

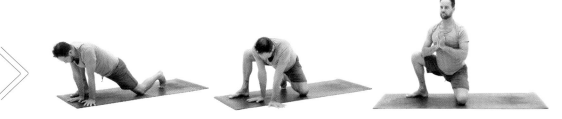

THAI STANCE TRANSITIONS

HALF TABLE (HT)

Step right foot forward, palm to the left

MONKEY (MO) PALMING

Draw left foot in, arms vertical, exhale to pour weight into hands

MONKEY (MO)

Sit hips on back heel, hands in prayer, *3 breaths*

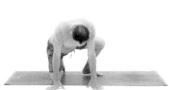

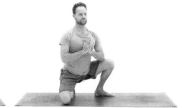

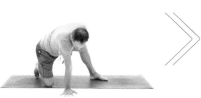

RUSSIAN DANCE

Switch sides: Hands to earth, lower right knee, raise left knee

MONKEY (MO)

Sit hips on back heel, hands in prayer, *3 breaths*

MONKEY (MO) PALMING

Palm toward right with straight arms

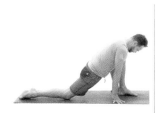

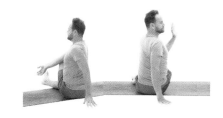

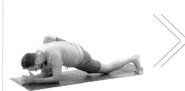

LOW LUNGE (LL)

Bend front knee, hips forward, chest up, *3 breaths*

SPINAL TWIST

Turn right and sit. Step left foot outside straight right leg, right arm outside left knee, *3 breaths*

Switch sides: Step right foot outside straight left leg, left arm outside right knee, *3 breaths*

LIZARD (Lz)

Step left leg back, hands or forearms to earth inside right foot, left leg extended, *3 breaths*

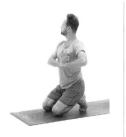

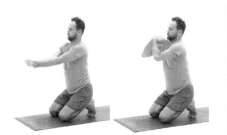

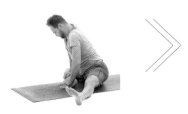

(Se) ARM STRETCH

Hands in prayer, inhale at center, exhale push palms to one side and look away, *3 breaths*. *Switch sides, 3 breaths*

(Se) WRIST ROLLS

Keeping wrists connected, circle wrists 3 times toward the body, then 3 times away

JANUSIRSASANA (Ja) SELF-MASSAGE

Sit with one leg straight, other leg bent. Palm and thumb the foot and calf of bent leg

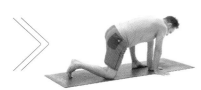

HALF TABLE (HT)

Finish palming with hands by left foot, swing right foot back

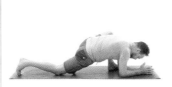

HIP & SPINE OPENING

LIZARD (Lz)

Hands or forearms to earth inside left foot, right leg extended, *3 breaths*

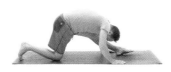

HALF SPLIT (1/2Sp)

Straighten front leg, shift hips back, relax head over front leg, *3 breaths*

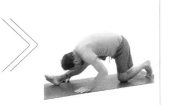

HALF SPLIT (1/2Sp)

Straighten front leg, shift hips back, relax head over front leg, *3 breaths*

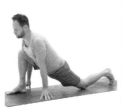

LOW LUNGE (LL)

Bend front knee, hips forward, chest up, *3 breaths*

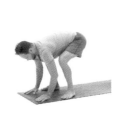

SUPPORTED SQUAT (Sq)

Step back foot forward, feet wide, knees bent, hands to earth, *3 breaths*

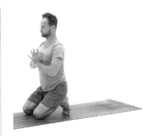

SELF CARE

SEIZA (Se)

Bring knees to the floor, keep all ten toes flexed and spread

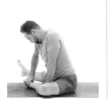

Switch sides and repeat thumbing and palming

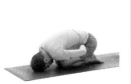

CHILD'S POSE (Ch) WITH FISTS

Sit onto tucked legs, fists to top of thighs. Fold over and breathe into stomach, *3 breaths*

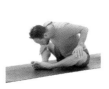

CLOSING

Bring feet forward, soles of feet touching, knees open to the side. Softly brush legs from thighs to toes. *Repeat 3 times*

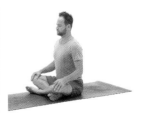

MEDITATION

Sit cross-legged with a tall spine, using a pillow if needed. *Seal in your practice for 1–10 minutes*

THAI MASSAGE

Thai massage is not from Thailand and is not just massage. Its roots are in Buddhism and Ayurvedic medicine that both come from India. The Buddha's message and ancient medical knowledge traveled from person to person, from border to border, and landed in Thailand centuries ago. There, in Thai monasteries, monks would meditate for hours on topics like loving-kindness, emptiness, suffering, and compassion, to name a few.

Here is where you can apply the wisdom gained from your self practice in the Lunar Asana Sequence.

When this physical practice is done with the spiritual seeds of compassion, loving-kindness, and zen-like presence, this treatment can affect more than just the body of the receiver.

Move slowly and stay receptive to your receiver's feedback.

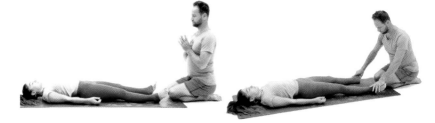

1. CENTERING

Sit in Hero (He) Pose with knees at your receiver's feet and hands in prayer. Rub your hands together to create heat.

2. FIRST TOUCH

Let warm hands land on your receiver's feet. Keep your mind clear and body still for a few moments as you connect with your receiver.

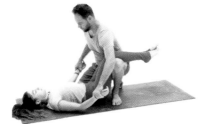

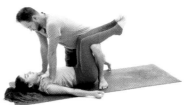

6. ARM HARMONICS

With their legs still draped, sit into Monkey Pose (Mo). Grasp their wrists and shake their arms to make waves in their upper body.

7. PALM SHOULDERS

Return to Half Table (HT), palm press one shoulder, then the other. Look for Perfect Fit of your palms on their shoulders.

After long sessions of sitting, their bodies would have aches and pains. Thai massage became a practice that brought the Buddhist principles to life through a moving meditation.

Based on the idea that there are energy lines in the body, Thai Massage is done fully clothed, on the ground, on a soft surface. By placing a receiver in different passive yoga poses and massaging these lines, you can promote the body's natural flow of circulation and healing potential.

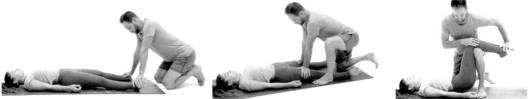
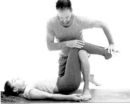

3. PALM FEET

Flex your feet to Seiza (Se), inhale lift one hand, exhale to place it on their foot and sink bodyweight through your straight vertical arm. *Alternate sides 4–6 times.*

4. PALM THIGHS

Step one foot forward to Half Table (HT), inhale lift one hand, exhale to place it on their thigh and sink bodyweight through your straight vertical arm. *Alternate sides 4–6 times.*

5. SACRAL FLOAT

Shift 90 degrees toward your grounded knee. In Half Kneeling (HK), drape the bend of their knees over your thigh. Push their feet down and rock their hips from side to side.

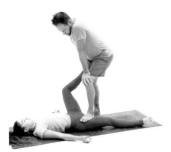
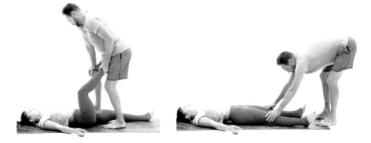

8. BLOOD STOP: LEFT FOOT

Hold their left heel and step your left foot diagonally on their other thigh. Sink bodyweight into their leg and feel for their pulse. *Hold for 30–60 seconds.*

9. BLOOD STOP: RIGHT FOOT

Repeat on the other leg. This technique is not to be used on people who are pregnant or have high or low blood pressure.

10. BRUSH LEGS

Softly brush their legs three times from hips to toes, feeling appreciation for the chance to practice listening and compassion.

THERAPEUTIC FLYING

Because of imbalances, injuries, stress, and the chaos of life, our bodies get misaligned. We spend most of our waking lives upright, resisting against gravity. Gravity is smarter than our beliefs of how we should sit, stand, or walk. When our body is inverted and relaxed on a skilled base's feet, our imbalances both new and old are invited back into balance. In just a few breaths, receivers can restore significant space between their vertebrae and reset their spine's orientation.

Therapuetic flights can range from two to twenty minutes, limited to or expanded by the base's ability to do flying transitions that change the position of the flyer. As the base gets more skilled they learn to address and touch many aspects of the receiver (skeletal, muscular, fascial, vascular, emotional). Flyers learn that they can be held and that they can trust, and this state helps them release their tensions and fears.

Once a therapeutic flight has been exchanged there exists an essence connection that forms a sturdy platform for friendship to grow. The wisdom gained in Thai massage is now brought into a three-dimensional flying playground. It is hard to put into words the transformational power of this aspect of AcroYoga practice. Therapeutic flying is the gem of therapeutics and if you dedicate yourself to it you will make lots of friends for life!

Therapeutic Flying Principles

BASES:
- » Keep legs stable, hands and feet soft.
- » Communicate clearly.
- » Be receptive.

FLYERS:
- » Ask for what you need.
- » Breathe deeply.
- » Relax and enjoy.

SPOTTERS:
- » Stand to the side.
- » Belly faces the center of gravity of the flyer.
- » Hands ready to support.

Lifted Butterfly (LB)

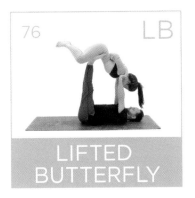

FOUNDATION: Hands under the front of the flyer's shoulders, feet turned out just below the flyer's hips supporting the flyer's thighs.

BASE ACTIONS: Bend legs to receive flyer's weight, place hands and feet to create the foundation, then extend arms and legs until either or both are vertical and straight.

FLYER ACTIONS: Lean into the base's support, then reach for wrists or forearms behind your back; bring feet into the butterfly shape and look for your feet, then relax.

BENEFITS: Gives a gentle traction to the spine; is very stable because there are four points of contact; the base and flyer are face to face so it is easy to communicate.

CHALLENGES: It can be hard for the base to find correct hand placement to create traction on the flyer's spine; base's feet can cause skin burn or rub on the flyer's hip bones.

Folded Leaf (FL)

FOUNDATION: Feet turned out, the inner edges of the base's feet touching the outer edges of the flyer's hip bones.

BASE ACTIONS: Bend legs to receive the flyer's weight, then extend legs until vertical.

FLYER ACTIONS: Place base's feet at your hips and lean into their support; relax, surrender, and let the legs come into a Piked Straddle (PiStr).

CHALLENGES: If the flyer is much taller than the base, flyer may have a hard time relaxing due to their head being compressed in the base's belly; it can be too intimate for some.

High Flying Whale (HFW)

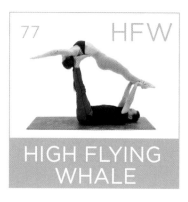

FOUNDATION: Heels between the spine and shoulder blades supporting the flyer's upper back; hands of the base supporting the ankles of the flyer.

BASE ACTIONS: Receive flyer's upper body, extend legs back past vertical, then straighten arms.

FLYER ACTIONS: From standing by the base's head, squat down and lay your upper body on their feet, adjusting the base's foot placement before going up. Lean back, look back, and communicate your needs to the spotter or base.

BENEFITS: Increases flyer's upper back mobility and boosts their energy; is accessible and enjoyable for many types of people; is very stable because there are four points of contact and the base does not need a lot of hamstring flexibility.

CHALLENGES: Can be a lot of extension on the flyer's neck; base's feet can be too hard or too pointed, creating discomfortable for the flyer.

VARIATIONS: Flyer's arms fully extended; hands interlaced behind the neck; arms crossed at the chest.

Reverse Prayer (RP)

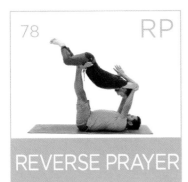

FOUNDATION: Base's feet turned out, inner edges of the base's feet touching the outer edges of the flyer's hip bones; flyer's elbows supported by the base's hands.

BASE ACTIONS: Keep arms and legs straight and support flyer's optimal elbow alignment.

FLYER ACTIONS: Place base's feet at your hips and lean into their support; bring elbows as close as is comfortable, breathe deeply, communicate your needs.

BENEFITS: Opens flyer's upper back, shoulders, and triceps.

CHALLENGES: Can injure flyer's shoulders if base moves flyer's arms abruptly while they are in deep flexion.

VARIATIONS: Flyers can widen the elbows or push down into the base to make the stretch less intense.

Walnut (Wa)

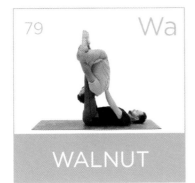

FOUNDATION: Feet turned out, inner edges of the base's feet touching the outer edges of the flyer's hip bones.

BASE ACTIONS: From Folded Leaf (FL), bend legs to create space for the flyer's head, then guide the flyer's head through your legs. Once through, straighten the legs; rock the legs toward your hands and massage the upper back and neck.

FLYER ACTIONS: Reach for your ankles outside the base's legs, point your toes up toward the ceiling, and tuck your chin to your chest as the base guides your head through.

BENEFITS: Flyer relaxation and release of upper back tension; good variation for flyers who are taller than their bases.

CHALLENGES: It can be too intimate; the head and ears can get squished between the base's legs; flyer must keep their feet pointed up to stay close to the base's support.

Back Leaf (BL)

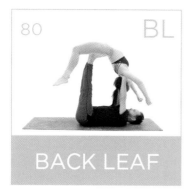

FOUNDATION: Base's feet turned out just below the flyer's gluteal fold.

BASE ACTIONS: Receive the flyer's weight by bending arms and legs until the flyer's center of gravity is over you, then extend both arms and legs vertical.

FLYER ACTIONS: From standing by the base's legs, lean back into the support of the base and relax.

BENEFITS: Very approachable; energizes the flyer.

CHALLENGES: Can be hard for bases to get their legs extended as they need to bend their knees deeply to reach the flyer's shoulders initially.

Bat (Bat)

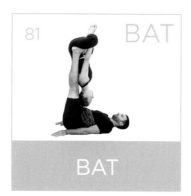

FOUNDATION: Base's feet parallel, inner edges of the base's feet touching the outer hip bones of the flyer.

BASE ACTIONS: From Back Leaf (BL), support the flyer's shoulders as they bring their legs into position; adjust your feet to be close to the flyer's hips.

FLYER ACTIONS: From Back Leaf (BL), hold the base's ankles, lean back, and bring your legs into a Piked Straddle (PiStr); then reach for your ankles, feet together with your toes pointed up.

SPOTTING: From the side; as the flyer gets their legs past vertical, move to the flyer's backside.

BENEFITS: One of the most versatile therapeutic poses; many back, neck, and shoulder release techniques can be used here.

CHALLENGES: If the flyer does not pike enough the base's feet slip away from the flyer's center.

FLY AND THAI

Back when Jenny and I started AcroYoga, we knew that Thai massage and therapeutic flying would be two elements of the practice, but it took us a while to figure out how to put them together. With time we came upon Fly & Thai, or a therapeutic AcroYoga flight paired with a Thai massage for the base, also called 'Leg Love.'

In therapeutic flights, the flyer receives lots of movement and opening in their upper body, and the base gets a leg workout. When the flyer comes down, they can offer a few simple moves to help the base's recovery and decompression, while getting a leg workout of their own! In this way both partners enjoy being active and receiving a treatment.

Since these two puzzle pieces have come together, Fly & Thai has revealed itself to be a beautiful ritual of giving and receiving, traction and compression, inhaling and exhaling, trusting and letting go.

The best part is that as you advance your knowledge of therapeutic flying transitions, your flyers will likely start having giggle fits in the air. When I give therapeutic flights I like to say that I get paid in giggles. When laughter becomes involved, everyone wins—the base, the flyer and anyone witnessing the joyful scene.

Forward Flying Level 1

» As the flyer, remember to breathe deeply and communicate how you feel so your base can best meet your needs.

» As the base, be receptive to your flyer's feedback and open to making adjustments.

Leg Love

» As the giver, move slowly and pay attention to your receiver's breath. Check in with them about how they feel.

» As the receiver, make sure you are comfortable. Breathe deeply, relax fully, and communicate if you need something to change.

Forward Flying Level 1

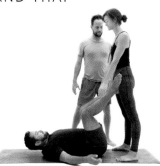

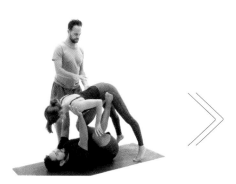

1. LIFTED BUTTERFLY (LB) PREP

Flyer stands close to base, placing their feet turned out below the flyer's hips. Flyer rests their hands on base's shins.

2. (LB) MOUNT

Flyer leans forward and base receives their weight by placing hands on flyer's shoulders and bending arms and legs.

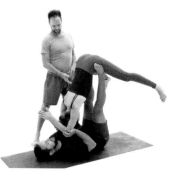

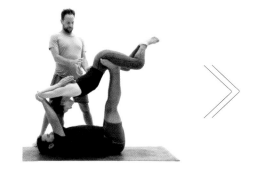

6. REVERSE PRAYER (RP) PREP

Flyer bends arms and base brings hands just below flyer's elbows. Base then straightens their arms.

7. REVERSE PRAYER (RP)

Flyer brings legs into Butterfly shape. Flyer's elbows can move together or apart depending on the stretch they want. *3 breaths*

'Leg Love' Thai Massage Sequence

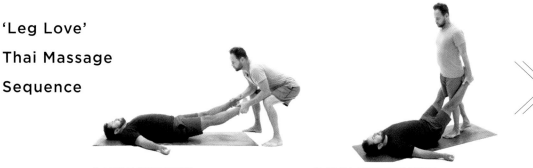

1. LEG HARMONICS

Holding their ankles, move base's feet quickly like windshield wipers, big toes pointing in and out, to loosen their legs and hips.

2. BULL FIGHTER PREP

Bring base's heels into your hands and hook their feet behind your hips by internally rotating their feet so their big toes come to touch. Inhale.

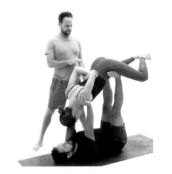

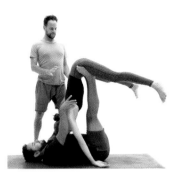

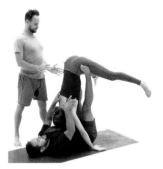

3. LIFTED BUTTERFLY (LB)

Base extends arms and legs vertically as flyer brings legs into Butterfly shape, wrists clasped behind their back. *3 breaths*

4. FOLDED LEAF (FL)

Flyer straightens legs to Piked Straddle as base bends their arms to lower flyer's head. Base lays backs of flyer's hands on the floor.

5. FOLDED LEAF (FL) MASSAGE

Base explores flyer's upper back, neck, shoulders, and arms by squeezing, palming and using thumbs to apply pressure. *3 breaths*

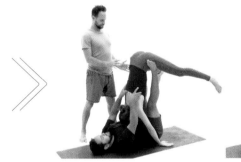

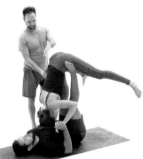

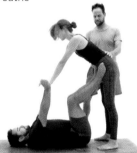

8. FOLDED LEAF (FL)

Flyer straightens legs to Piked Straddle as base lowers flyer's head. Base lays backs of flyer's hands on the floor. *3 breaths*

9. PREPARE TO LAND

Partners take a Reverse Hand to Hand Grip and take a deep inhale together.

10. LANDING

Both partners straighten arms, base bends their legs, and flyer settles feet back to the ground.

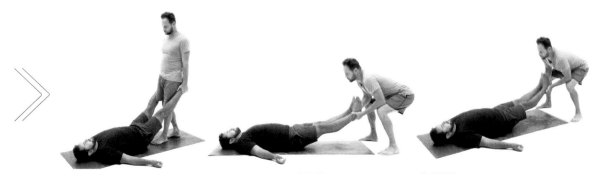

3. BULL FIGHTER

Exhale as you lean your weight back to create traction in base's legs, hips, and spine. Repeat three times.

4. SPINAL ROCKS

Squat wide with your forearms on your thighs. Lean forward and back slowly or quickly to create traction and compression in their spine.

5. FISH

Bring base's feet together and move them from side to side like a fish tail. Slowly lower legs to the ground to close Leg Love.

17

THE SUSTAINABLE WAY

A long life may not be good enough, but a good life is long enough.
—BENJAMIN FRANKLIN

In this quote Mr. Franklin speaks to how we value the quality of our time versus the quantity of our time. For me they are both important and related. If you train in a way that is aligned with your passions and interests, you are already winning—this is quality time. If you know what you want to keep learning and growing throughout your whole life, you are addressing your quantity of time.

To get far in life and in AcroYoga, we have to play the long game of sustainability. The Sustainable Way is the safest way to reach high levels in any practice, and it is the only way you can keep doing them for the rest of your life. There are some skills in acrobatics that took me over ten years of dedication just to taste my first few seconds of success. Basing a standing, extended, one-arm hand to hand was this unicorn-type skill. To get there, I had to balance quantity of training with quality by integrating the

principles I will describe in this chapter.

My concepts of sustainability were synthesized through observing and working with those who embody them. I am privileged to witness many different kinds of talented individuals from all over the world—from countless disciplines, tall to small, super strong to crazy flexible. Out of this variety I have a special place in my heart for the humble masters sixty years of age and older. There are four masters in particular whose stories I want to share. These people are lit up by what they do, and they love to help others get better. They are brutally honest and in service of destroying excess ego. They make fun of typical human mental traps. Their embodiment is light, but deep, skilled, and precise.

The first master I met was George Nissen, the inventor of trampolines. Before I ever met him, I already knew I loved this man because I loved his invention. At my first sports acrobatics national championship in Riverside, California in 1988, I saw George, in his nineties at the time, jump into a one-minute handstand at the awards ceremony, right at the table where he was sitting! Witnessing this moment taught me that if you choose to incorporate movement into your daily routine, you can keep your mobility and your joy throughout your entire life. Part of how we age rests on our beliefs and the accumulation of our daily habits.

In 2001 I met the second master, Sri Dharma Mittra, who became my guru and taught me about spiritual connection through practicing devotional *asana*. He says things like, "Every *asana* is an offering to the Lord," and, "Most of yoga is learning how to control what goes in and comes out of your mouth." His 'how' is teaching yoga asana with yogic spiritual philosophy. His 'why' is spreading non-violence through a vegetarian diet and "being nice to everyone." At eighty-one years old, he still does roughly 25 percent of every yoga class he teaches at the Dharma Yoga Center in the heart of Manhattan. His classes almost always include a headstand with no hands, and he holds it longer than all the students there! He moves with more fluidity and grace than most humans I have met. Dharma

eats mainly raw vegan food and is 100 percent committed to sharing his passion for yoga as a path of purification and self-knowledge.

The third of these four masters was Lu Yi. A Chinese circus master, he was in his sixties when I met him in San Francisco at the world-renowned Circus Center in 2003. He had rituals and routines that kept him very able-bodied into his mid-seventies. He did five sets of twenty push-ups and five one-minute handstands against the wall every day. He would also, with his fists, strike the outsides of his legs daily and sip on his mason jar filled with water and green tea leaves. His routines were incredibly fixed. Because of this, he could do and teach things that had never crossed my mind. One day, I came into the circus center and watched him teach a child how to sit on the handlebars of a bike and peddle it facing the back tire. In my own practice, he taught me more about handstands than any one person I've worked with. How he unlocked my handstand potential was simple: we did not train new skills; we trained new levels of precision and deeper levels of humility in the same skills. For years our routine, just like his own, was fixed: one two-minute handstand, one set of ten press handstands (straddle and pike), four sets of one-arm handstands, two sets of handstand-to-one-arm levers, and after each set he would stretch me in a hollow pike to balance my strength with my flexibility. Once in a blue moon we would try a new leg variation, but our routine training offered plenty of room to grow my subtle awareness and eventually unlock my one-arm handstands.

The fourth master I met was Arjun Pichet Aon Phawat Boonthumme, in 2008. Pichet is a spiritual teacher from Thailand who is deeply steeped in Buddhism and Thai massage. To study with him you need to arrive at eight a.m. with flowers, candles, 800 baht (about 25 US dollars), and leave your ego at the door. Humility is a prerequisite. After students place their offerings at the altar, everyone chants Buddhist mantras while sitting on flexed toes for twenty minutes straight. He then gives and receives Thai massage for the whole day. His body is so open and relaxed due to years of his dedicated practices that he is able to fall asleep in some of the strangest yoga positions. Imagine sitting with your shins against the floor and your butt between your feet, then lying back. This pose is called *supta virasana,* and while I experience emotional and physical tantrums when I do this pose, he snores in it! He is always laughing and

making fun of life while teaching Buddhist philosophy. One of his classic lines is about attachment and suffering: "Oh, I think, I like, I want . . . big headache!" He goes on laughing. One of his gifts is being dedicated to his *dharma*, or path, and sharing his passion with the *sanga,* or community. He is a living master—a wellspring of ancient wisdom in a modern world. He teaches his students how to be lazy yet effective Thai massage therapists while at the same time inviting them deeper into their own spiritual paths.

As these masters demonstrate, you can really practice yoga, acrobatics, and therapeutics for your whole life, and this is one of the many things I love about all three roots of AcroYoga. We grow old when we stop believing we can do things and when we say we are too old to do things. What these four masters have in common is they know what they are passionate about, and their passion has a through line from body and mind to emotions and spirit. Their mastery is infused with joy and a lightheartedness that makes their practices flow with ease. The average person will most likely not master any of these arts, but we can dedicate our lives to learning and enjoying the ride.

I realize that many of my master teachers have been men. As sustainability and balance are two means to the same end, with the presentation of this book and my experiences comes the acknowledgment that for my life's work to be more sustainable, I will be seeking out more women to learn from in the second half of my life. To that point, I want to recognize my mother and grandmothers for being my greatest teachers about life, love, and ultimately about being human.

RECOVERY TRAINING

Recovery is vital to progress, growth, and sustainability. As a general premise, for whatever body region or modality you've trained hard, you should do something that either contrasts that modality or rests that area. For example, after standing acrobatics and handstands, which put a lot of weight on the wrists and forearms, we focus on releasing compression from those parts of the body. This basic principle can help anyone balance the way they train.

At the end of strong physical training, the body is very warm, so flexibility gains can increase substantially during this time. Self-massage is key to understanding your body and, in time, to applying that wisdom to healing others. Foam rolling is a very lonely yet effective way to get more blood and nutrients to the tissues to help them recover, and to bring more elasticity or flexibility to an area. You will know you are doing recovery right if you feel good at the end of your practice and you addressed the parts of your body that you worked hard during the solar exercises.

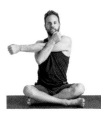 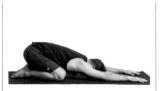 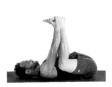 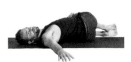

ARM STRETCH

» Bring one arm across your chest and use the other arm to stretch into the shoulder.

» Great to do after practices that use upper body strength.

CHILD'S POSE (CH)

» Sit on your shins with knees together or wide and arms outstretched.

» Helpful after inversions; stretches the ankles and shoulders, opens the lower back, and massages the internal organs.

HAPPY BABY

» Lie on your back with legs up and bent and reach for your big toes or outer edges of the feet.

» Beneficial at the end of any movement practice; opens feet, hips, and lower back.

RECLINED SPINAL TWIST

» Lie on your back with knees up and legs bent, then swing knees to one side and look the other way.

» Useful at the beginning or end of day; creates space between the vertebra and massages the internal organs.

SELF-CARE

Remember, if you ever need a helping hand, it's at the end of your arm.
—AUDREY HEPBURN

As much as AcroYoga is a practice of partnership and connection, it will never take the place of you helping yourself. In fact, the more depth we have in our relationships the more important it is to come back to ourselves and take moments for self-care and self-love.

I have yet to find a language whose word for "selfish" does not have a negative connotation. Yet ultimately, being "selfish" is at the core of how we can give to others. When our cup is full, we have more to share. On some level, we are the ideal person to offer support to ourselves as we are the ones constantly receiving signals from our own bodies, giving us clues as to our true needs and desires.

When we practice self-care, we are aiming towards rejuvenation. This word spells out why we do these practices. *Juve*, like juvenile, refers to youth; *re* means "again," and *ate* indicates "to make," as in "to make young again." You can think of self-care like taking your car in for a tune-up. Whatever fluids are low, you fill; whatever is out of alignment, you get back into place. The tune-ups you need will depend on how you use your car and where its imbalances lie. Sometimes all you need is to wash the car and put on a coat of wax. Self-care by definition is not a dreadful process—it is just the opposite. Self-care is doing what makes you feel better and what you need to balance your mind, body, or emotions. Ideally you enjoy doing it in the moment, and without a doubt you enjoy the aftereffects.

Playfulness and laughter are central to AcroYoga, and there are many other ways we can bring vitality into our lives each time we practice. It's about small, daily investments in health and happiness versus a weekend binging on a spa package. These practices help us fill our cup again and again so we are set up well for our next activities. Here is a short list of ideas you might try:

SELF-CARE IDEAS
» self-massage *(see Lunar Asana pg 264)*
» warm baths
» taking naps
» walks in nature
» talking to friends
» reading & journaling
» meditation
» listening to or playing music
» saunas & cold plunging
» playing with animals or children
» eating yummy, nourishing food

NOBLE ELEMENTS OF SUSTAINABILITY

These are the three Noble Elements at the top of the AcroYoga Table of Elements. They are not the best, but they are the most subtle and can be very easily lost as life and emotions break us out of these delicate states of being. The first step is to touch these places and see for yourself what their effects are on your life and your relationships. Chances are, as you value these states more you will dedicate yourself to spending more time there.

Presence (Pr)

63 Pr
PRESENCE

When the theoretical mind shuts down and the physical practices take over all of you in one moment, this is the power of being present. Acrobats spend so much of their time in the present moment because they have to in order to stay safe. Their practices take them to new edges each time they train. In therapeutics, as you touch one part of the body with full presence, you find a greater capacity to sense the rest of the body as a whole.

The present is a specific point in the timeline between past and future. Your mind can be in different places along that line; what will serve you depends on the situation. It is thanks to our big brains that we can live in these different paradigms.

To maximize happiness it is vital to sharpen your awareness of what percentage of your day you spend in each of these dimensions. Past and future have gifts of insight and direction and can expand your potential to dream and integrate. Their power is valid, but they will never be as tangible as the present moment. Everything real happens in the present moment. When someone is fully present with us, they are able to give us all of their magic.

Compassion (Cp)

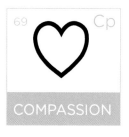

The root of "compassion" comes from the Latin word *compassus,* meaning "co-suffering"; it is our ability to relate to others' suffering. Accessibility is a powerful attribute of compassion—you need no special training, degrees, or language to access it. All people have access to it because we all feel and we all suffer. As our awareness of our own suffering increases, we can grow our desire to be compassionate toward others.

Practicing compassion can greatly improve our quality of life by helping us move from judgment to acceptance. With years of dedicated practice, we can accept and love more people. With little work done here, we can become overly critical and feel separate from people. As our compassion grows, the ability to connect to bigger groups of people expands.

When this Noble Element takes root in your being, your speech, your touch, and the way you look at people will be wrapped in this sweet, kind energy. You have nothing to lose by extending compassion to others, and when you grow this capacity, you tap into the potential to open your heart and change people's lives. Once this level of practice is consistent you will have learned the most important tool for building community and supporting the well-being of those around you.

Peace (Pe)

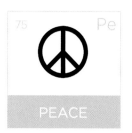

Peace is a tender state that is supported by realizing that as human beings we all suffer and we all will die. The Buddha became enlightened when he was sitting under the bodhi tree with his spine pressed against it. In this moment he felt so safe and protected by the tree that he let go of his fears and attachments. Peace rides along the river from attachment to non-attachment. A non-attached state is in harmony with the reality that we are transient, and posessions do not come with us after we leave our bodies.

A lot of our human suffering is caught up in our attachments to what we want and what we fear losing. You might like your partner to stay longer in skills and not give up so easily. When your peace is dependent on what others give you or do not give you, your peace will always be fleeting. What really deserves your stress and anxiety?

As you become more present to the gift that life is, and have compassion for yourself and others, peace can begin to expand within you. Peace is like perfection; they are both moving targets and destinations. They are like light—a wave and a particle, a probability and a singularity. It's easy to be at peace in a day spa, but when you can be at peace while someone is threatening or offending you, you know you are a deep practitioner.

SEALING IN THE GOODNESS

Even if you never read this section, simply by doing AcroYoga you would develop these qualities by trial and error. If you dedicate yourself to cultivating the physical elements in the AcroYoga Table of Elements, the Noble Elements will naturally begin to blossom in your life and manifest in your relationships.

Now that you have planted the seeds, you are well on your way toward seeing and feeling the true depths of practice possible in AcroYoga. To make these theories more applicable, on the next pages are five principles you can keep as little coaches on your shoulder as you build your sustainable AcroYoga practice.

SUSTAINABLE TRAINING PRINCIPLES

1. Train Smart, Not Hard.

AcroYoga is designed to be a lifelong practice, and efficiency will always win over time. Fewer attempts with more skill will produce better results in the long run than mindless repetitions with hazardous falls. If your body is healthy and happy, this is one sign that you are training smart. If you find yourself injured often, you could be doing too much of a good thing!

The quality of your interactions with your partners, spotters, and teachers is also key to smart training. If you are angry, not grounded, or reactionary with your partners, or if they are like this with you, your AcroYoga practice will be very taxing and draining. Co-creating a positive training environment is the sustainable way forward.

2. Cultivate Gratitude, Contentment, and Patience.

It is likely in life and in AcroYoga that you will experience difficulty and suffer injuries. In this state we can feel sad, frustrated, and even angry that we cannot do what we could before. When the emotional storm settles, there is always wisdom to be found in our new, modified bodies. We can be grateful for all the parts of us that work well, content with the game of making new modifications to our practice, and patient in the healing process.

Daily gratitude rituals can provide a steady way to balance the reality that life is not always fun. Being grateful and not needing more, or practicing contentment, is a powerhouse combination. I find these states in meditation; while sitting quietly, I realize I don't need much, and what I do need I already have.

After gratitude and contentment, patience is the third hero. Patience is not complacency; it is clearing space in your mind and heart to grow in the direction of your dreams. It takes time to build your practice and your partnerships, but each step can be celebrated. Rome was not built in a day. Continue progressing in your skills while being careful not to go so fast that you forget to enjoy the ride.

3. To Go Fast, Go Alone; to Go Far, Go Together.

Speed is not a determining factor in the quality or depth of your relationships. Going fast and achieving skills are very important things for many of us. But if this is the primary way you engage with AcroYoga, you will end up with very few friends (and you need friends to do AcroYoga!)

You never know who will be the one to show you something pivotal and unexpected in your AcroYoga journey. Slowing down and moving with others in mind will make your practice more rich, and you will find more resources to get what you want, and what you didn't know you needed, from AcroYoga and from life.

4. Find Your Teacher.

The student-teacher relationship is one of the oldest and most deeply valuable of all human relationships. It pays to be selective with your teachers, as they will help you establish your habits. Good habits set a wise, stable foundation on which to build your practice. Inefficient backyard techniques, or bad habits, take double the time to re-pattern down the road.

When you find a teacher you trust, open your mind to what they have to share. Receive their teachings as truth, and build upon them by testing their theories in your own practices. If something does not make sense, ask more questions.

You should not have to give up who you are to dedicate

yourself to a discipline. If you find the right teacher, they will want you to keep who you are and at the same time they will teach you the structure you need to develop your practice. The right education will feed you for life.

5. Know Your 'Why.'

The four masters I mentioned at the beginning of this chapter knew their purpose on this earth and have lived in harmony with that knowing. I think of the 'why' like a nuclear reactor: with just a bit of input you can generate enormous amounts of energy.

How did Serena Willams win 23 Grand Slam singles titles, the most by any man or woman? How, at age forty two, did Kareem Abdul-Jabbar retire with the title of NBA's all-time leader in points scored (38,387)? How did Jennifer Lee, writer and director of *Frozen* and *Frozen II,* earn an Academy Award for Best Animated Feature, becoming the first female director of a feature film that earned more than $1 billion in gross box office revenue?

When you know your 'why,' you can always find more inspiration and energy to reach your goals. Ideally, training is something you do because you enjoy it and the benefits it brings to your life. There are so many things we must do as adults because we are told to or feel we should. I believe my success as an athlete came primarily from doing it because I loved it. If you don't love it, find something else that you do love.

From there, be curious and find people who know more than you do about what you are training. Ask questions and listen deeply. Finding your 'why' can be a slippery fish, because we are human and we change our minds often. A good sign of you being on your path to distilling your 'why' is when time vanishes, focus is easy, and magic happens. If you want long-term success with anything you do in life, your 'why' is the spark that will keep your fire lit.

"True freedom is living in the present moment, where the gratitude for what is exceeds the desire for what might be."

—GURU SINGH

SUSTAINABILITY JOURNALING
REFLECT & CLARIFY YOUR SUSTAINABLE PATH

Sustainability Journaling is a practice that can unite your current desires with the long-term effects of your decisions and actions.

AcroYoga is designed to be accessible throughout all the stages of your life, and this journaling prompt can help you assess how you want the years ahead to look for you.

The answers you distill in response to these questions can serve as a powerful guiding light in how you go forward moving through life. When you have some time to reflect, sit down with a pen and paper and answer the following questions.

Outward Reflection
1. Write the name of someone you know who is older than you and does AcroYoga (or another similar movement practice).
2. What do you observe about the way they train or practice? What inspires you about them?
3. Of those observations, what would you like to integrate into your own life?

Inward Reflection
4. What qualities or elements do I enjoy the most about my practice?
5. Where do I regularly struggle in my practice?
6. Which skills or practices do I want to keep doing for my whole life?
7. Which skills do I think I won't do for my whole life, and why not?

Make a Path Forward
8. What qualities or exercises can I dedicate to that will support the longevity of my training?
9. What self-care am I already doing that works well for me? What new self-care activities would I like to try?

As an example, your Sustainability Journaling might look something like this:

1. *Det.*
2. *She is very joyful in her training, and she knows what to say 'no' to.*
3. *I want to copy-paste her energy into my training—I want to really enjoy my training, and get comfortable with saying 'no' to things that will hurt my body.*
4. *I love helping others reach new skills. I love making people giggle when I fly them.*
5. *I have not had a regular training partner for a few years and that makes my acro practice less interesting for me.*
6. *Handstands, therapeutic flying, and Thai massage are all practices I know I want to keep doing for my whole life.*
7. *As some point I think my joints will not want to sustain the force of some high impact activities like running and tumbling.*
8. *To support the longevity of my training I can practice patience, using smart progressions, and being more consistent with doing some movement every day.*
9. *I take baths almost every morning. I would like to add more self-massage with oil. I want to do this at least once a week.*

VISIT *WWW.ACROYOGA.ORG/MCP* TO DOWNLOAD A FREE WORKBOOK, WATCH TUTORIALS, AND FIND OUR COMPANION VIDEO COURSE TO HELP YOU ACTIVATE THE PRINCIPLES AND PRACTICES DISCUSSED IN THIS CHAPTER.

THE FUTURE I SEE: MOVING FORWARD TOGETHER

Our health rests on us using our bodies in the ways for which they were designed. It's a theory you have seen before, and it's part of my mission of movement, connection, and play: We must use it not to lose it. In order to grow our movement potential, we must keep testing our bodies in new ways and moving every day. To maintain connection with ourselves, we must listen to the signals our bodies give us in response to our lifestyles and our choices. To grow our connections with others, we must continue investing in our friendships and showing up for those we love. And for play to be a part of our lives forever, we must continually allow ourselves to let go, laugh, and have fun.

While we are alive we can move our bodies, our breath, and our friends. Even if you sit at work for eight hours per day, movement, connection, and play can still be a reality for you, and eventually it can become your new norm. Play reveals our inner child, a part of us that can always remind us how fun and happy life can be, and community keeps us supported in the face of the predictable struggles we all face in life. When we are connected to a community of fun-loving, kind, and talented movers, shakers, and healers we get lifted emotionally and physically. This is the goal I see in front of us as a species, and the good news is that with the tools in this book it is not hard to reach. When the pieces of our life are balanced, we can exist in a bountiful state of peace that affects everything we do and everyone we meet. The better we get at filling our cup and feeling joy, the more possible it becomes to give more to others. When our love and awareness expand from ourselves to our families, friends, and eventually strangers, we will know what yogis call oneness, what Jamacians call "One Love," and what I call us reaching our true potential as human beings.

ACKNOWLEDGMENTS

There are not enough pages in this book to thank all the people who have helped make *Move, Connect, Play* a reality. First and foremost I thank my mother, Katie, for being my first teacher and biggest support throughout my life; my father, Tony, for teaching me about Mexican culture *güey* and being a steady business advisor for AcroYoga International; my stepfather, John, for being my first shaman, healer, and wizard of many types of magic; my stepmother, Nancy, for teaching me old world and Canadian culture; my grandma and *abuelita* for showing me two very different ways to love unconditionally; and all of my family, living and passed, who have shaped my worldview and given me many of the tools that make me who I am today.

Thank you to Jenny Sauer-Klein for being an amazing partner in crime, co-teacher, and co-founder as we birthed AcroYoga into the world. To Sri Dharma Mittra, I am eternally grateful for the spiritual teachings and insights you shared with me in unlocking the mystical world of yoga. Lu Yi, your teachings will forever echo around the AcroYoga community; thank you for sharing your decades of Chinese circus wisdom with me and always emphasizing the value of human connection.

These acknowledgments would not be complete without recognizing Jessie Goldberg and Eugene Poku, the founders of AcroYoga Montreal, as trailblazers on the path to sharing different and complementary forms of movement, connection, and play. And to the Thai Circus family, thank you for opening my mind to how fun, creative, and connective the healing arts can be.

Britta Rael, without your support this book would never have seen the light of day; your rock-steady friendship and full spectrum of talent are why people are reading these words now. Nayef Zarrour, your advice has helped me become a more centered and conscious man, and your input helped this book become more inclusive and far-reaching. Erin O'Halloran, your ability to ask me the right questions and your courage to reorganize the whole book hurricane-style made an invaluable contribution. Katie Veleta, you were the master seamstress who helped to thread this book together; your insight on yoga and neuroscience was priceless.

Aaron Alexander, thank you for introducing me to my agent, Jaidree Braddix. Jaidree, thank you for helping me to dream big. Daniela Rapp, you were the only editor who said yes to a first flight as we pitched this book deal; our flow has been fun and full of trust since that first leap. And to Rising McDowell, your passion, dedication, and attention to detail turned this book into a beautiful and useful work of art that I am so proud of, and that will bring immense value to all who read it. I will forever cherish your love toward me and this project.

I also offer deep, deep gratitude to Tim Ferriss and B. Tim, your mentorship and enthusiasm for AcroYoga has opened so many doors for me and the practice; B., your desire to learn and grow pushed me to develop new ways to organize and teach AcroYoga. During the beginning of the 2020 pandemic, your zoomed-in, smiling faces were the only ones I saw as this book was being written; thank you for your friendship and dedication to strengthening your practice and relationship through AcroYoga.

To all the AcroYogis who have taken the steps to become a certified teacher and have literally uplifted thousands of new AcroYogis, my respect and gratitude for you is immense. Lastly, I extend my thanks to every person who has invited AcroYoga into their life. Because of you, what started out as a couple of friends playing in a park in San Francisco has blossomed into a beautiful global family where there are no strangers.

INDEX